Study Guide
Cooper & Gosnell

Adult Health Nursing

Eighth Edition

Candice Kumagai

Formerly Instructor in Clinical Nursing
University of Texas at Austin
Austin, Texas

ELSEVIER

ELSEVIER

3251 Riverport Lane
St. Louis, Missouri 63043

STUDY GUIDE FOR ADULT HEALTH NURSING, Eighth edition ISBN: 978-0-323-52387-5

Notices

Content Strategist: Nancy O'Brien
Senior Content Development Specialist: Diane Chatman
Publishing Services Manager: Jeff Patterson
Project Manager: Carol O'Connell
Design Direction: Renee Duenow

Printed in United States of America

Last digit is the print number: 9 8 7 6 5 4 3 2

Working together
to grow libraries in
developing countries

www.elsevier.com • www.bookaid.org

To the Student

Understanding fundamental concepts and principles of nursing will prepare you for patient care experiences. By mastering the content of your *Adult Health Nursing* textbook, you will have the necessary knowledge and skills for nursing practice. This Study Guide was created to help you achieve the objectives of each chapter in the textbook, establish a solid base of knowledge in the fundamentals of nursing, and evaluate your understanding of this critical information.

Each Study Guide chapter is organized into sections, each with its own topic and related objectives from the textbook. Different types of learning activities, including short answer, multiple choice, table activities, matching, and figure labeling, assist you in meeting these content objectives. To maximize the benefits of this Study Guide and prepare for the learning activities:

1. Carefully read the chapter in the textbook and highlight, note, or outline important information.
2. Review the Key Points, access the Additional Learning Resources, and complete the Review Questions for the NCLEX® Examination at the end of each textbook chapter.
3. Complete the Study Guide exercises to the best of your ability.
4. Time and pace yourself during the completion of each exercise. You should spend approximately 1 minute for each multiple choice and matching question, and approximately 2 minutes for completion activities or short answer questions.
5. After completing an exercise, refer to the textbook page references as needed. You can then repeat any exercises for additional practice and review. A complete Answer Key is provided on the Evolve Resources website.

ADDITIONAL LEARNING RESOURCES

Additional Learning Resources are available on the Evolve website at http://evolve.elsevier.com/Cooper/adult/.

Evolve

- Review Questions for the NCLEX® Examination (for each chapter)
- Answer Key for all Study Guide questions
- Calculators
- Fluids and Electrolytes Tutorial
- Immunization Schedule
- Spanish/English Glossary
- Additional Animations
- Additional Audio Clips
- Additional Video Clips
- Skills Performance Checklists
- Body Spectrum Electronic Anatomy Coloring Book

STUDY HINTS FOR ALL STUDENTS

- *Ask questions!* There are no bad questions. If you do not know something or are not sure, you need to find out. Other people may be wondering the same thing but may be too shy to ask. The answer could mean life or death to your patient, which certainly is more important than feeling embarrassed about asking a question.
- *Make use of chapter objectives.* At the beginning of each chapter in the textbook are objectives that you should have mastered when you finished studying that chapter. Write these objectives in your notebook, leaving a blank space after each. Fill in the answers as you find them while reading the chapter. Review to make sure your answers are correct and complete, and use these answers when you study for tests. This should also be done for separate course objectives that your instructor has listed in your class syllabus.

- *Locate and understand key terms.* At the beginning of each chapter in the textbook are key terms that you will encounter as you read the chapter. Page numbers are provided for easy reference and review, and the key terms are in bold, blue font the first time they appear in the chapter. Phonetic pronunciations are provided for terms that might be difficult to pronounce.
- *Review Key Points.* Use the Key Points at the end of each chapter in the textbook to help you review for exams.
- *Get the most from your textbook.* When reading each chapter in the textbook, look at the subject headings to learn what each section is about. Read first for the general meaning, then reread parts you did not understand. It may help to read those parts aloud. Carefully read the information given in each table and study each figure and its caption.
- *Follow up on difficult concepts.* While studying, put difficult concepts into your own words to see if you understand them. Check this understanding with another student or the instructor. Write these in your notebook.
- *Take useful notes.* When taking lecture notes in class, leave a large margin on the left side of each notebook page and write only on right-hand pages, leaving all left-hand pages blank. Look over your lecture notes soon after each class, while your memory is fresh. Fill in missing words, complete sentences and ideas, and underline key phrases, definitions, and concepts. At the top of each page, write the topic of that page. In the left margin, write the key word for that part of your notes. On the opposite left-hand page, write a summary or outline that combines material from both the textbook and the lecture. These can be your study notes for review.
- *Join or form a study group.* Form a study group with some other students so you can help one another. Practice speaking and reading aloud, ask questions about material you are not sure about, and work together to find answers.
- *Improve your study skills.* Good study skills are essential for achieving your goals in nursing. Time management, efficient use of study time, and a consistent approach to studying are all beneficial. There are various study methods for reading a textbook and for taking class notes. Some methods that have proven helpful can be found in *Saunders Student Nurse Planner: A Guide to Success in Nursing School* by Susan C. deWit. This book contains helpful information on test-taking and preparing for clinical experiences. It includes an example of a "time map" for planning study time and a blank form that you can use to formulate a personal time map.

ADDITIONAL STUDY HINTS FOR STUDENTS WHO USE ENGLISH AS A SECOND LANGUAGE (ESL)

- *Find a first-language buddy.* ESL students should find a first-language buddy—another student who is a native speaker of English and is willing to answer questions about word meanings, pronunciations, and culture. Maybe your buddy would like to learn about your language and culture. This could help in his or her nursing experience as well.
- *Expand your vocabulary.* If you find a nontechnical word you do not know (e.g., *drowsy*), try to guess its meaning from the sentence (e.g., *With electrolyte imbalance, the patient may feel fatigued and drowsy*). If you are not sure of the meaning, or if it seems particularly important, look it up in the dictionary.
- *Keep a vocabulary notebook.* Keep a small alphabetized notebook or address book in which you can write down new nontechnical words you read or hear along with their meanings and pronunciations. Write each word under its initial letter so you can find it easily, as in a dictionary. For words you do not know or for words that have a different meaning in nursing, write down how they are used and sound. Look up their meanings in a dictionary or ask your instructor or first-language buddy. Then write the different meanings or usages that you have found in your book, including the nursing meaning. Continue to add new words as you discover them. For example:
  - *Primary*—Of most importance; main (e.g., *the primary problem or disease*); The first one; elementary (e.g., *primary school*)
  - *Secondary*—Of less importance; resulting from another problem or disease (e.g., *a secondary symptom*); The second one (e.g., *secondary school* ["high school" in the United States])

Illustration Credits

Chapter 1
P. 2: Harkreader H, Hogan MA, & Thobaben M: *Fundamentals of nursing: Caring and clinical judgment*, ed 3, St. Louis, 2007, Saunders.

Chapter 3
P. 16: Patton KT & Thibodeau GA: *The human body in health and disease*, ed 7, St. Louis, 2018, Elsevier.

Chapter 4
P. 23: Patton KT & Thibodeau GA: *The human body in health and disease*, ed 7, St. Louis, 2018, Elsevier.

Chapter 5
P. 29: Thibodeau GA & Patton KT: *Anatomy and physiology*, ed 10, St. Louis, 2019, Mosby.

Chapter 8
P. 49: Canobbio M: *Mosby's clinical nursing series: Cardiovascular disorders*, St. Louis, 1990, Mosby.

Chapter 11
P. 76: Patton KT & Thibodeau GA: *Anatomy and physiology*, ed 8, St. Louis, 2013, Mosby.

Chapter 12
P. 83: Thibodeau GA & Patton KT: *Structure and function of the body*, ed 14, St. Louis, 2012, Mosby.
P. 85: Seidel HM, Ball JW, Dains JE, et al.: *Mosby's guide to physical examination*, ed 7, St. Louis, 2011, Mosby.

Chapter 13
P. 93: Patton KT & Thibodeau GA: *Anatomy and physiology*, ed 10, St. Louis, 2019, Elsevier.
P. 94: Patton KT & Thibodeau GA: *The human body in health and disease*, ed 7, St. Louis, 2018, Elsevier.

Chapter 14
P. 101: Patton KT & Thibodeau GA: *The human body in health and disease*, ed 7, St. Louis, 2018, Elsevier.
P. 102: Ignatavicius DD, Workman ML, Blair M, et al: *Medical-surgical nursing: Patient-centered collaborative care*, ed 8, St. Louis, 2016, Elsevier.

Chapter 15
P. 111: Grimes D: *Infectious diseases*, St. Louis, 1991, Mosby.

Introduction to Anatomy and Physiology

Answer Key: Textbook page references are provided as a guide for answering these questions. A complete Answer Key is provided in your Additional Learning Resources on Evolve.

CROSSWORD PUZZLE

1. Directions: Use the clues to complete the crossword puzzle.

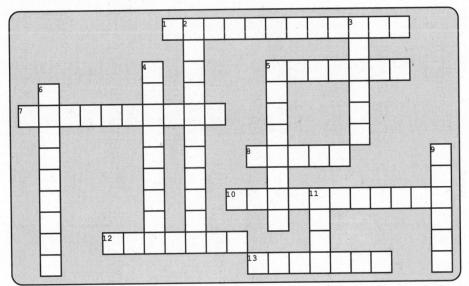

Across

1. Engulf and digest foreign material *(7)*
5. Cell division *(6)*
7. Movement of water and particles through a membrane by force from either pressure or gravity *(8)*
8. Several kinds of tissues united to perform a more complex function *(11)*
10. Extracellular fluid taken into the cell and digested *(7)*
12. Diffusion of water through a selectively permeable membrane in the presence of at least one impermeant solute *(8)*
13. Largest organelle within the cell *(5)*

Down

2. Body's internal environment is relatively constant *(4)*
3. Perform more complex functions than any one organ can perform alone *(4)*
4. Internal living material of cells *(5)*
5. Thin sheets of tissue that serve many functions in the body *(9)*
6. Solid particles in a fluid move from an area of higher concentration to an area of lower concentration *(8)*
9. Groups of similar cells that work together to perform a specific function *(8)*
11. Smallest living unit of structure and function in the body *(12)*

FIGURE LABELING

Planes of the Body

2. Directions: Label the figure below with the correct names of the body planes and anatomical directionality of the body: sagittal, coronal, ventral, dorsal, transverse, caudal, and cranial. *(2)*

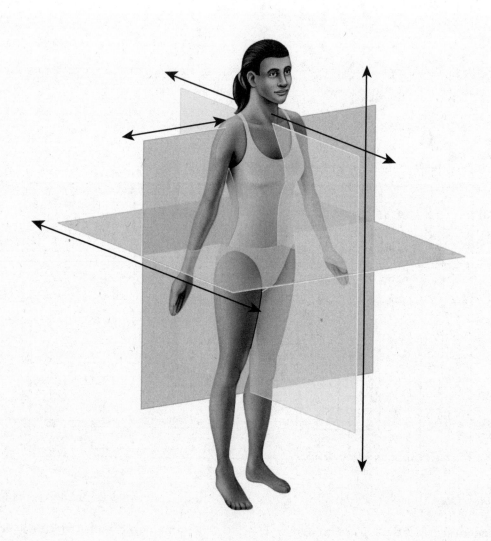

TABLE ACTIVITY

3. The table below lists one part of each of the major systems of the body. Identify the major system and then identify at least one function. *(11)*

One Body Part of Major System	Major System	Function
Lungs		
Blood vessels		
Brain		
Stomach		
Kidneys		
Bones		
Voluntary muscles		
Skin		
Thyroid gland		
Lymph nodes		
Gonads		

MULTIPLE CHOICE

Directions: Select the best answer(s) for each of the following questions.

4. The patient reports, "I ran into the coffee table and bruised my shin." Which sample of documentation **best** reflects the nurse's knowledge of anatomy and medical terminology? *(1)*
   1. Skin damage noted on the right lower leg in the shin area
   2. Patient reports running into coffee table and bruising shin
   3. Moderate bruising noted on the patient's right leg just below knee
   4. 4-cm ecchymosis on mid-anterior of right tibia-fibula

5. The patient needs assistance to turn and move in bed and is at risk for the complications of immobility. The nurse documents with date and signature: 10:00 Assisted into a right lateral side-lying position; 12:00 Assisted into supine position; 14:00 Assisted into left lateral side-lying position. What is the **best** rationale for this type of documentation? *(1)*
   1. Documentation shows that needs were met and the goal was achieved.
   2. Documentation reflects actions taken to prevent complications of immobility.
   3. Nurse is following standard documentation guidelines.
   4. Nurse is demonstrating a professional knowledge of terminology.

6. The nurse reads in the chart that the neglected infant sustained a superficial sunburn on the dorsal body surface. What instructions would the nurse give to the unlicensed assistive personnel? *(1)*
   1. "You will see a thin film of cream on the baby's perineal area."
   2. "If you see peeling or blistering on the front of the chest, let me know."
   3. "Use tepid water and gently wash the baby's back and pat dry."
   4. "The baby's face and the top of his head may appear red and flaky."

7. The nurse is checking peripheral pulses on a patient who has peripheral vascular disease. Which pulse is the **most** distal in the lower extremities? *(2)*
   1. Dorsalis pedis
   2. Popliteal
   3. Posterior tibial
   4. Femoral

8. Which anatomical structure is in the medial portion of the chest? *(1)*
   1. Lungs
   2. Heart
   3. Sternum
   4. Clavicles

9. Which part of the cell has distinct surface proteins that play an important role in tissue typing to determine compatibility for organ transplant? *(5)*
   1. Protoplasm
   2. Nucleus
   3. Cytoplasm
   4. Plasma membrane

10. One type of cell in the body relies on the action of the ion pump to move nearly all calcium ions to special compartments or out of the cell. What bodily function is **most** affected by this process? *(8)*
    1. Muscle contraction
    2. Digestion of food
    3. Protection against infection
    4. Secretion of hormones

11. The health care provider tells the nurse that the patient has a hematopoietic disorder. Which laboratory result would the nurse expect to see? *(10)*
    1. Decreased potassium
    2. Decreased red blood cell count
    3. Increased glucose
    4. Increased blood urea nitrogen

12. For a patient with a history of splenectomy, which topic is the nurse **most** likely to review to ensure that the patient has a good understanding of the self-care related to loss of the spleen? *(11)*
    1. Blood glucose monitoring
    2. Dietary sources of fiber
    3. Infection control measures
    4. Fall prevention

13. The patient reports pain in the right upper abdomen just inferior to the ribs. Based on the nurse's knowledge of anatomy, which organ is **most** likely to be contributing to the patient's discomfort? *(3)*
    1. Small intestine
    2. Spleen
    3. Gallbladder
    4. Cecum

14. The nurse suspects that the patient has urinary retention and must assess for bladder distention. Which region of the patient's abdomen will the nurse palpate? *(3)*
    1. Umbilical region
    2. Hypogastric region
    3. Right hypochondriac region
    4. Left iliac region

15. The patient has a stomach ulcer. Based on knowledge of anatomy, the nurse recognizes that the patient is likely to report pain or discomfort in which region of the abdomen? *(3)*
    1. Epigastric region
    2. Right iliac region
    3. Left lumbar region
    4. Hypogastric region

16. The patient is diagnosed with appendicitis. The health care provider orders ice to the abdomen pending emergency surgery. Where will the nurse place the prepared ice bag? *(4)*
    1. Left lower quadrant
    2. Right lower quadrant
    3. Left upper quadrant
    4. Right upper quadrant

17. In the case of bowel obstruction, which condition is **most** likely to cause the first episodes of vomiting if the patient is consuming solid foods? *(4)*
    1. Distal large intestine obstruction
    2. Proximal large intestine obstruction
    3. Distal small intestine obstruction
    4. Proximal small intestine obstruction

18. The patient sustains injury to the epidermis. Which problem will the nurse anticipate and try to prevent? *(10, 11)*
    1. Risk for infection
    2. Loss of strength
    3. Decreased secretion of mucus
    4. Loss of insulation

19. The patient is in a coma and has continuous open-mouthed breathing, which causes dry mucous membranes of the mouth. What is the **most** important rationale for the nurse to perform good oral hygiene for this patient? *(11)*
    1. Preserve patient's dignity
    2. Lubricate food for digestion
    3. Prevent respiratory infection
    4. Maintain condition of teeth

20. The patient tells the nurse that he has a history of bursitis. Which focused assessment is the nurse **most** likely to perform that relates to this information? *(11)*
    1. Auscultate the bowel sounds and palpate the abdomen.
    2. Auscultate the lung sounds and watch respiratory effort.
    3. Put joints through range of motion and ask about discomfort.
    4. Ask patient to balance on right leg and then on left leg.

CRITICAL THINKING ACTIVITIES

Activity 1

21. Why is it important for the nurse to have knowledge of anatomy and physiology? *(1)* _____

_____

_____

_____

_____

Activity 2

22. The patient says, "I have a bruise on the tip of my right big toe." Document the patient's report using anatomical terminology. *(1)*

_____

_____

_____

_____

_____

Activity 3

23. Discuss how the accurate usage and correct spelling of anatomical terminology enhances the credibility of your nursing documentation. *(1)*

_____

_____

_____

_____

_____

Care of the Surgical Patient

Answer Key: Textbook page references are provided as a guide for answering these questions. A complete Answer Key is provided in your Additional Learning Resources on Evolve.

TABLE ACTIVITY

1. Directions: The patient has just returned from gastric surgery. Next to each assessment, list normal findings and the frequency of data collection. *(43, 44, 45, 48, 49, 50)*

Assessment	Normal Findings	Frequency
a. Vital signs		
b. Incision		
c. Respiratory effort		
d. Pain		
e. Urinary function		
f. Neurovascular		
g. Activity		
h. Gastrointestinal function		

MATCHING

Directions: Match the term or suffix on the left with the meaning on the right. (16)

Term	Meaning
_____ 2. anastomosis	a. Surgical removal of
_____ 3. -ectomy	b. Direct visualization by a scope
_____ 4. -lysis	c. Opening into
_____ 5. -orrhaphy	d. Surgical joining of two ducts or blood vessels to allow flow from one to another; to bypass an area
_____ 6. -oscopy	e. Surgical repair of
_____ 7. -ostomy	f. Destruction or dissolution of
_____ 8. -otomy	g. Opening made to allow the passage of drainage
_____ 9. -pexy	h. Plastic surgery
_____ 10. -plasty	i. Fixation of

MULTIPLE CHOICE

Directions: Select the best answer(s) for each of the following questions.

11. After surgery, which foods would the nurse suggest to the patient that are specific for building and repairing body tissue? *(18)*
    1. Variety of foods but avoid processed sugar
    2. Lean meat and low-fat dairy products
    3. Whole grain breads and cereals
    4. Seasonal fruits and leafy green vegetables

12. The newly hired nurse is told that generally morning medications are withheld on the day of surgery. The nurse is **most** likely to clarify withholding which medication? *(20)*
    1. Phenytoin
    2. Warfarin sodium
    3. Ranitidine
    4. Acetaminophen

13. Which preoperative patient teaching topics are a nursing responsibility? **Select all that apply.** *(19)*
    1. Gastrointestinal cleansing preparation
    2. Need for assistive devices postoperatively (e.g., crutches)
    3. Date and time of the surgery
    4. Risks and benefits of the procedure
    5. Written pre- and postoperative instructions

14. The nurse is reviewing the presurgical laboratory results for a patient who has a history of cardiac problems. Which abnormal result is of **greatest** concern? *(23)*
    1. Sodium: 146 mEq/L
    2. Blood glucose: 130 mg/dL
    3. Blood urea nitrogen: 25 mg/dL
    4. Potassium: 5.8 mEq/L

15. The nurse is interviewing the patient to obtain a medical history prior to a surgical procedure. Which patient report warrants further investigation because of a possible latex allergy? *(25)*
    1. Had sore throat after having a nasogastric tube inserted for stomach decompression
    2. Developed a large hematoma in the antecubital fossa after donating blood
    3. Experienced severe swelling of the labia after urinary catheterization
    4. Had skin irritation after dermabrasion to remove a small precancerous growth

16. Which data set is **most** important to note prior to starting the skin preparation before surgery? *(25)*
    1. Temperature, turgor, and dryness of skin; history of dehydration and electrolyte imbalance
    2. Presence of infection, irritation, bruises, or lesions on skin; history of skin allergies
    3. Underlying structures such as veins, arteries, or nerves; history of peripheral vascular disease
    4. Color of skin, sensation to touch, and hair distribution; history of peripheral neuropathy

17. The patient is in the postanesthesia care unit and is having difficulty maintaining a patent airway after extubation. Which intervention would be used to maintain a patent airway until the patient is fully conscious? *(37)*
    1. Ventilate using a bag-valve-mask
    2. Use an oral suction catheter
    3. Give oxygen per nasal cannula
    4. Insert an oral airway

18. What is the significance of the nurse's signature on the preoperative checklist? *(39)*
    1. Specifies that the preoperative medication was given
    2. Delegates care on the list to the appropriate staff members
    3. Indicates the nurse assumes responsibility for care on the list
    4. Confirms that the patient understands the preoperative care

19. What postoperative assessments would the nurse make to comply with the facility policy based on the "times 4" factor? *(44)*
    1. Takes vital signs, checks IV, incisional sites, and any tubes 4 times every hour for 4 hours, then every hour times 4 hours, then every 4 hours times 4 days
    2. Does vital signs and general assessments every 15 minutes times 4 (for 4 times), every 30 minutes times 4, every hour times 4, then every 4 hours
    3. Takes pulse, blood pressure, respiratory rate, and pulse oximeter readings every 15 minutes times 4 (for 4 times), then every hour until assessments approximate baseline
    4. Does vital signs, checks IV, incisional sites, tubes, and postoperative orders every 15 minutes times 4 (for 4 times), then delegates vital signs every hour times 4 hours

20. The postsurgical patient manifests hypotension; tachycardia; restlessness; apprehension; and cold, moist, pale skin. How does the nurse interpret these findings and what action would the nurse take **first**? *(45)*
    1. Suspects hypoglycemia and administers IV 10% dextrose per standard protocol
    2. Suspects a panic attack and administers a PRN (as needed) dose of lorazepam
    3. Suspects airway obstruction and inserts an oral airway using nursing judgment
    4. Suspects hypovolemic shock and administers oxygen per standard protocol

21. The patient is in the induction stage of anesthesia. Which activity will **most** likely be taking place? *(37)*
    1. Positioning the patient to perform the surgical procedure
    2. Decreasing the dosage of anesthetic agents
    3. Cleaning, shaving, and preparing the skin
    4. Establishing and verifying placement of the endotracheal tube

22. During the preoperative teaching session, a patient voices concerns about waking up during surgery. Which response should the nurse give to the patient? *(37)*
    1. "The anesthesia given during surgery will not wear off and allow you to wake up."
    2. "The anesthesiologist is able to monitor for this and will provide medications as needed."
    3. "There is a very small chance of waking towards the end of the surgical procedure."
    4. "Don't be concerned; emergence from anesthesia is very rare."

23. The patient is scheduled to undergo a urologic procedure in the surgical suite. The patient will be conscious during the procedure. What type of anesthesia will **most** likely be used? *(37)*
    1. Nerve block
    2. Epidural anesthesia
    3. Spinal anesthesia
    4. Local anesthesia

24. The patient is scheduled to undergo the removal of a benign cyst from his hand in the health care provider's office. The nurse is aware that the provider will **most** likely use which type of anesthesia? *(38)*
    1. Regional anesthesia
    2. Local anesthesia
    3. Moderate sedation
    4. Intrathecal anesthesia

25. The nurse is preparing to assist the surgeon who is performing a procedure using moderate sedation. Which nursing action is the **most** important during the procedure? *(38)*
    1. Monitoring intake and output
    2. Administering the medication
    3. Reassuring the patient
    4. Assessing vital signs

26. The nurse is preparing an in-service for nursing staff about moderate sedation. What should be emphasized in the presentation? *(39)*
    1. There will be temporary paralysis and loss of sensation in the legs.
    2. There is a risk of aspiration and laryngeal spasm after extubation.
    3. Resuscitation equipment should be readily available.
    4. Patients have a risk for thrombus because of prolonged positioning.

27. When developing the plan of care for an Arab American undergoing surgery, what is a cultural consideration? *(20)*
    1. Stoicism during pain and discomfort
    2. Expected submissive role of women
    3. Need for a written consent for surgery
    4. Avoidance of sustained eye contact

28. When is the **best** time to perform preoperative teaching? *(20, 22)*
    1. 1 to 2 days before surgery
    2. Morning of surgery
    3. At least 2 weeks preoperatively
    4. When the nurse has extra time

29. Before surgery on the bowel, what is the purpose of administering neomycin, sulfonamides, or erythromycin? *(23)*
    1. Decreases likelihood of bowel perforation
    2. Prevents urinary tract infections
    3. Detoxifies the gastrointestinal tract
    4. Reduces the risk of pneumonia

30. The nurse is providing care for a patient in the postanesthesia care unit after emergency surgery. The patient has been on antihypertensive medications for a long time. What side effects related to use of these medications should the nurse monitor for? *(36)*
    1. Bradypnea
    2. Hypotension
    3. Tachycardia
    4. Diaphoresis

31. The patient is instructed to discontinue taking nonsteroidal antiinflammatory drugs (NSAIDs) for several days before surgery. What is the **best** explanation for the need to hold this medication? *(36)*
    1. "NSAIDs increase susceptibility to postoperative bleeding."
    2. "NSAIDs impair healing during the postoperative period."
    3. "NSAIDs interact with the medications used for anesthesia."
    4. "NSAIDs are associated with an increase in postoperative infections."

32. A mastectomy is scheduled for an 81-year-old patient. What is the **highest** priority during the immediate postoperative recovery period? *(44)*
    1. Assessing for confusion
    2. Airway management
    3. Pain management
    4. Monitoring bleeding

33. The patient is being prepared to go to the operating room. With proper instructions, which tasks can be delegated to the unlicensed assistive personnel (UAP)? **Select all that apply.** *(17)*
    1. Compare current vital signs to baseline measurements.
    2. Assist the patient to remove personal clothing and don a hospital gown.
    3. Check the IV pump rate and the IV insertion site.
    4. Assist the patient to move from the bed to the stretcher.
    5. Ensure that the preoperative checklist is complete.
    6. Apply antiembolic stockings.

34. The nurse is performing preoperative teaching for a patient who must undergo a breast biopsy. The patient begins to cry softly and says, "I can't believe this is happening to me." What response should the nurse use **first**? *(18)*
    1. "Do you need more information about the procedure?"
    2. "The biopsy is a minor procedure, there are very few risks."
    3. "Don't worry, everything will be okay; we'll take care of you."
    4. "You seem scared; tell me what you are thinking about."

35. Which patient is **most** likely to have problems related to medications that are given in the perioperative setting? *(18)*
    1. A 23-year-old woman who believes in alternative and complementary therapies
    2. A 73-year-old woman who takes multiple medications for several chronic conditions
    3. A 56-year-old man who has recently started an oral antidiabetic medication
    4. A 7-year-old child who occasionally uses a rescue inhaler for asthma

36. The patient tells the nurse that he has been smoking for years and is likely to continue to smoke before and after his surgery. Which piece of equipment will the nurse emphasize during the preoperative teaching? *(20)*
    1. Normal range for pulse oximeter
    2. Use of incentive spirometer
    3. Use of patient-controlled analgesia pump
    4. Operation of the call bell

37. The nurse is evaluating the patient's understanding of the preoperative teaching. Which question should the nurse ask? *(21)*
    1. "Do you have any questions about the postoperative care?"
    2. "Would you like written information about the care plan?"
    3. "Did you understand everything I told you about the care?"
    4. "What questions do you have about the postoperative care?"

38. The surgeon is preparing to explain a procedure to the patient and obtain informed consent. Which information is the **most** vital to relate to the surgeon before he/she enters the patient's room? *(23)*
    1. Patient has been talking about refusing the surgery.
    2. Patient had a hypoglycemic episode 3 hours ago.
    3. Patient's laboratory reports are not available yet.
    4. Patient received morphine and a sedative 1 hour ago.

39. The patient is to have nothing by mouth (NPO) starting at midnight the night before surgery. Which task can be delegated to the UAP? *(23)*
    1. Give the patient small sips of water if he reports thirst.
    2. Assist with oral care, but instruct the patient not to swallow fluids.
    3. Obtain small hard candy for the patient to suck on.
    4. Check the patient's intravenous fluids every 2 hours.

40. Which patient should not be instructed to cough after surgery? *(28)*
    1. The patient who had abdominal surgery
    2. The patient who had pneumonia before surgery
    3. The patient who had intracranial surgery
    4. The patient who had thoracic surgery

41. The patient had surgery at 10:00 AM. At 6:00 PM, the nurse notes that the patient has not voided since returning from surgery. What should the nurse do **first**? *(48)*
    1. Help the patient to the toilet and open the faucet so that water runs.
    2. Palpate the symphysis pubis to determine if the bladder is distended.
    3. Call the surgeon and obtain an order for catheterization.
    4. Help the patient get up and ambulate to stimulate urination.

42. The patient is undergoing spinal anesthesia and the patient's position has to be slightly adjusted during the procedure. Which occurrence is cause for **greatest** concern? *(37)*
    1. Slight decrease in blood pressure
    2. Loss of sensation in both feet
    3. Slowing of respiratory rate
    4. Inability to freely move the legs

43. A patient who had surgery on the left hip tells the nurse, "You might think I am crazy, but my right arm kind of hurts since I had my surgery." What should the nurse do **first**? *(39)*
    1. Check the operating records for patient's position during the operation.
    2. Call the surgeon and inform him/her of the new-onset arm pain.
    3. Assess the arm for pulse, sensation, movement, pain, and temperature of skin.
    4. Give the patient a mild pain medication and elevate the arm on a pillow.

44. Which instruction is the nurse **most** likely to give to the patient before administering the preoperative medication? *(39)*
    1. "Please go to the bathroom and void."
    2. "Let me mark the operative site."
    3. "I am going to draw a blood sample."
    4. "Please sign the consent form."

45. The patient will soon be transferred from the postanesthesia care unit to the nursing unit. Which tasks can be delegated to the UAP? **Select all that apply.** *(17)*
    1. Place the bed in a high position with side rails in appropriate position.
    2. Obtain a clean gown and extra pillows for positioning.
    3. Set up suction equipment and test function.
    4. Get stethoscope, thermometer, and sphygmomanometer.
    5. Check the function of the IV pump.
    6. Place bed pads to protect linens from drainage.

46. The anesthesiologist has written the order to transfer the patient from the postanesthesia care unit to the nursing unit. Which assessment finding would delay the transfer? *(43)*
    1. Patient is awake, but nausea and some vomiting continue.
    2. Patient is breathing normally, but reports a sore throat and cough.
    3. Patient is crying and reports pain related to the surgical incision.
    4. Patient has a decreased blood pressure and pulse is increasing.

47. The patient had surgery 10 hours ago. The UAP tells the nurse that the blood pressure (BP) is 96/60 mm Hg and the patient says, "My blood pressure is usually 120/78." What should the nurse do **first**? *(45)*
    1. Check the patient for signs and symptoms of hypovolemic shock.
    2. Tell the UAP to go back and repeat the BP and report back.
    3. Tell the UAP to take and report BP and pulse every 5 minutes for 15 minutes.
    4. Call the surgeon and report the low reading of 96/60.

48. Which task is the responsibility of the scrub nurse? *(43)*
    1. Sends for the patient at the proper time
    2. Checks medical record for completeness
    3. Performs and confirms patient assessment
    4. Assists with surgical draping of patient

49. The nurse is preparing to discharge a patient from an ambulatory surgery setting. How does the nurse determine when the patient is ready to be discharged? *(53)*
    1. Patient states he is ready to drive himself home.
    2. Patient is groggy, but readily arouses to normal stimuli.
    3. Patient reports that pain is controlled and nausea has ceased.
    4. Family is available and willing to take responsibility.

50. The nurse is caring for a postoperative patient who has preexisting type 2 diabetes. Which assessment is **most** relevant to a complication associated with diabetes? *(18)*
    1. Impaired communication
    2. Bloody emesis
    3. Poor wound healing
    4. Hypoventilation

CRITICAL THINKING ACTIVITIES

Activity 1

51. Discuss latex allergies. Include types, influencing factors, risk factors, and methods of preventing problems for patients who have latex allergies. *(25)*

_____

_____

_____

_____

_____

_____

_____

Activity 2

52. Describe how the nurse can use the ABCDEF mnemonic device to ascertain serious illness or trauma in the preoperative patient. *(18)*

_____

_____

_____

_____

_____

_____

_____

Activity 3

53. Discuss four or five considerations for older adults who require surgery. *(18)* _____

_____

_____

_____

_____

_____

Care of the Patient With an Integumentary Disorder

chapter

3

Answer Key: Textbook page references are provided as a guide for answering these questions. A complete Answer Key is provided in your Additional Learning Resources on Evolve.

SHORT ANSWER

Directions: Using your own words, answer each question in the space provided.

1. What are the functions of the skin? *(56, 57)* _____

   _____

   _____

   _____

   _____

2. When performing an assessment of an integumentary problem, what should be included using "PQRST"? *(64)*

   _____

   _____

   _____

   _____

   _____

3. When performing an assessment of a mole, what characteristics should be included using "ABCDE" for assessment of skin lesions? *(64)*

   _____

   _____

   _____

   _____

   _____

4. The nurse is assessing the skin of several patients. What are the physiologic factors that influence skin color? *(59)*

    _____

    _____

5. The patient is a very dark-skinned individual who has low hemoglobin and hematocrit. How would the nurse assess this patient for pallor? *(64)*

    _____

6. The darker-skinned patient reports an itching sensation, but the nurse cannot detect a rash with visual inspection. What technique can the nurse use? *(64)*

    _____

FIGURE LABELING

Rule of Nines

7. Directions: Label the body according to the rule of nines. *(95)*

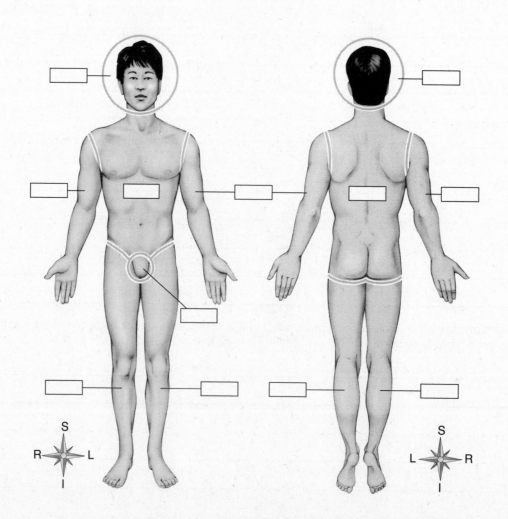

8. Calculate the percentage of burns for each of the situations listed below using the rule of nines. *(94, 95)*

   a. A 19-year-old was burned while playing with fireworks. He has burns on both of his arms (anterior and posterior) and his anterior chest and abdomen. _____%

   b. A 70-year-old man was burned when he backed up into an open-flame heater. He has burns on the posterior of his body from his ankles to his neck. He also has burns on the anterior portion of his legs. _____%

   c. The patient, who has diabetes mellitus, stepped into a hot shower and has burns on his back and buttocks. _____%

MULTIPLE CHOICE

Directions: Select the best answer(s) for each of the following questions

9. The nurse hears in report that the patient has anemia. Based on this information, what would the nurse expect to observe when assessing the patient's integumentary system? *(59)*
   1. Cyanosis in the periphery
   2. Yellow tinge of conjunctivae
   3. Pallor of mucous membranes
   4. Brown concentration of melanin

10. What would be considered **early** signs/symptoms of a pressure injury (Stage 1)? *(65)*
    1. Shallow, open, shiny, dry injury; pink-red wound bed without sloughing or bruising
    2. Full-thickness tissue loss, subcutaneous fat visible; possible undermining and tunneling
    3. Full-thickness tissue loss, slough and black eschar in wound bed with undermining and tunneling
    4. Intact skin with nonblanchable redness, painful, warm, soft localized area over a bony prominence

11. Which neonate has the **greatest** risk of being infected by herpes virus during childbirth? *(66)*
    1. Mother has chronic genital herpes, but was never treated.
    2. Mother contracted genital herpes during first half of pregnancy.
    3. Mother previously had severe genital herpes outbreaks.
    4. Mother acquired genital herpes near the time of delivery.

12. A patient is prescribed oral acyclovir for type 1 herpes simplex virus. What is the expected outcome if the patient is compliant with the medication regimen? *(68)*
    1. Prevents complications, such as meningitis or pneumonitis
    2. Shortens the outbreak and lessens the severity of symptoms
    3. Eliminates the likelihood of spreading the infection to others
    4. Decreases the probability of recurrent outbreaks

13. Which people have the **greatest** risk for serious complications secondary to herpes zoster infection? **Select all that apply.** *(73)*
    1. Healthy middle-aged adult who never had chickenpox
    2. Older adult who takes large doses of prednisone for a chronic condition
    3. Middle-aged adult who just started taking chemotherapy
    4. Nurse who recently received the first dose of varicella vaccine
    5. Young adult who is positive for the human immunodeficiency virus

14. The nurse must assess several patients who have skin disorders. Which disorder can manifest signs/symptoms that could be mistaken for venous thrombosis? *(74)*
    1. Cellulitis
    2. Pityriasis rosea
    3. Spider angioma
    4. Tinea corporis

15. What is the common factor for etiology and pathophysiology of folliculitis, furuncles, and carbuncles? *(75, 76)*
    1. Superficial infections are caused by fungus.
    2. Parasites get underneath the skin.
    3. Hair follicles are infected or inflamed.
    4. There is an allergic response to an allergen.

16. Which question would the nurse ask to assist the health care provider to determine the cause of contact dermatitis? *(78)*
    1. "Have you used any new soaps or detergents?"
    2. "Are you currently sexually active?"
    3. "Is anyone in the household having similar symptoms?"
    4. "Have you had a recent febrile illness?"

17. The patient comes to the walk-in clinic and reports noticing itching shortly after eating shrimp. The nurse observes that the patient has wheals over the anterior neck and chest. Which assessment would the nurse perform **first**? *(80)*
    1. Check orientation and observe for change in mental status.
    2. Auscultate heart sounds for pericardial friction rub.
    3. Take vital signs and observe for hypovolemic shock.
    4. Count respiratory rate and auscultate breath sounds.

18. The nurse instructs the patient on use of lindane. What additional instructions will the nurse give? *(88)*
    1. If skin lesion starts to bleed or ooze or feels different (swollen, hard, lumpy, itchy, or tender to the touch), report symptoms to the health care provider.
    2. Apply broad-spectrum sunscreens with a sun protection factor of 15 or greater approximately 15 minutes before sun exposure and after swimming.
    3. Furniture, carpeting, and car interiors must be cleaned. Wash bed linens in hot water; then use dryer. Put stuffed toys in hot dryer for a full cycle.
    4. Use neutral soaps and avoid hot water and vigorous rubbing. Skin and hair should be washed to remove excess oil and excretions and to prevent odor.

19. Which data set represents the signs/symptoms of an exacerbation of systemic lupus erythematosus? *(86)*
    1. Vesicles preceded by pain, generally in the thoracic region
    2. Fever, rash, cough, or increasing muscle and joint pain
    3. Erythema, pain, and tenderness over an area of skin
    4. Vesicles appear, ulcerate, rupture, and encrust

20. The nurse hears in report that a young female patient is very upset because of alopecia; she cannot focus on the overall cancer treatment plan. In addition to therapeutic communication, which intervention could the nurse use? *(92)*
    1. Suggest therapeutic baths using colloid solution.
    2. Teach the patient about use of scarves or wigs.
    3. Suggest shaving, tweezing, or rubbing with pumice.
    4. Advise the patient to use lotion immediately after bathing.

21. The health care provider has diagnosed a patient with paronychia. Which assessment is the nurse **most** likely to perform before administering the ordered therapy? *(93)*
    1. History of allergies to antibiotics
    2. Rating of pain on a pain scale
    3. Baseline range of motion
    4. Feelings about body image

22. A patient reports hair loss (hypotrichosis). Which assessment is the nurse **most** likely to conduct to assist the health care provider to determine the etiology of hypotrichosis? *(93)*
    1. Type of hair-care products
    2. Use of herbal supplements
    3. Smoking history
    4. Dietary assessment

23. A patient is admitted for pain and tenderness in his lower right leg. The nurse's assessment reveals that the extremity is warm, swollen, and has a slightly pitted appearance. Which measure would the nurse use to relieve the discomfort? *(74)*
    1. Assist the patient to ambulate as much as possible.
    2. Administer cool compresses or a covered ice bag.
    3. Elevate the leg with pillows to reduce edema.
    4. Assist with a therapeutic bath and gently pat skin to dry.

24. The nurse is assisting a mother to plan meals for a child who was recently diagnosed with eczema. Which foods should the nurse mention as common allergens associated with eczema? *(80)*
    1. Strawberries and cured meats
    2. Eggs, rye, and preservatives
    3. Orange juice, wheat, and eggs
    4. Wheat, sugar, and bananas

25. The nurse knows that the health care provider frequently prescribes isotretinoin for patients with acne. Which question is the **most** important to routinely ask? *(69)*
    1. "Are you pregnant or contemplating a pregnancy in the near future?"
    2. "Do you have a history of kidney problems or frequent urinary tract infections?"
    3. "How often do you sunbathe? Are you willing to abstain during treatment?"
    4. "Do you have any problems with your liver or a history of hepatitis?"

26. The nurse is interviewing an older adult. Which statement is cause for the **greatest** concern? *(90)*
    1. "My toenails are tough and thick."
    2. "This black mole on my neck is itching."
    3. "My hair is thinning and I have a bald spot."
    4. "I have a lot of 'age spots' on my hands."

27. The nurse notes that the patient has clubbing of the fingertips. Based on this finding, which question would the nurse ask? *(64)*
    1. "Have you been diagnosed with a respiratory disorder?"
    2. "Do you take medication for high blood pressure?"
    3. "Do you have a family history of diabetes mellitus?"
    4. "Are you taking medication for osteoporosis?"

28. To assess the temperature and texture of the patient's skin, which technique would the nurse use? *(64)*
    1. Use the fingertips and gently palpate the affected area.
    2. Use the palms of the hands and compare opposite body areas.
    3. Use a cotton-tipped applicator and apply gentle pressure.
    4. Use a gloved finger to touch skin and ask about sensations.

29. The school nurse is assessing a 15-year-old girl and notices multiple linear superficial cuts over the girl's anterior forearms. What should the nurse do **first**? *(64)*
    1. Call child protective services to report possible abuse.
    2. Notify the girl's parents about the finding.
    3. Ask the girl directly what happened to her arms.
    4. Initiate protective measures to prevent self-harm.

30. The nurse is assessing a patient who was recently transferred from home to a skilled nursing facility. The nurse sees a pressure injury with full-thickness tissue loss, which is covered by a thick, black layer of eschar. What should the nurse do **first**? *(65, 66)*
    1. Gently remove the eschar and check for tunneling and depth.
    2. Document the size and location of this stage IV injury.
    3. Contact the wound care specialist for wound management.
    4. Leave eschar intact; collaborate with RN to develop care plan.

31. The home health aide phones the nurse and says, "Yesterday, I helped the patient bathe. I wore gloves during the bath, but then afterwards he said that he was just diagnosed with herpes zoster." Which question would the nurse ask **first**? *(71, 72)*
    1. "Are you having a painful burning rash with itching?"
    2. "Did the patient have fluid-filled vesicles on the back or trunk?"
    3. "Have you received two doses of varicella vaccine?"
    4. "How long were you in contact with the patient?"

32. The nurse hears during shift report that the patient was admitted for penicillin-induced dermatitis medicamentosa. Which question is the **most** important to ask? *(79)*
    1. Was the affected area immediately washed and rinsed?
    2. Has the patient been medicated for pain and itching?
    3. Has the patient had any respiratory distress?
    4. Does the patient have any fever or other signs of infection?

33. The nurse would be prepared to administer epinephrine as needed for which patient? *(80)*
    1. Has burning sensation and a dry crusty lesion on the lip
    2. Has a single pink, scaly patch that resembles a large ringworm
    3. Has skin maceration, fissures, and vesicles around the toes
    4. Has raised red wheals and hives and an expiratory wheeze

CRITICAL THINKING ACTIVITIES

Activity 1

34. Discuss the nursing care of a patient who has sustained a major burn through the emergent phase, acute phase, and rehabilitation phase. *(96-100)*

    a. Emergent phase:_____

    _____

    _____

    b. Acute phase: _____

    _____

    _____

    c. Rehabilitation phase:_____

    _____

    _____

Activity 2

35. Discuss teaching points for self-examination of skin, scalp, moles, blemishes, and birthmarks. *(91)*

_____

_____

_____

_____

_____

_____

_____

36. Discuss teaching points for skin cancer prevention. *(91)* _____

_____

_____

_____

_____

_____

_____

_____

Care of the Patient With a Musculoskeletal Disorder

Answer Key: Textbook page references are provided as a guide for answering these questions. A complete Answer Key is provided in your Additional Learning Resources on Evolve.

FIGURE LABELING

1. Directions: Label the figure of the anterior view of skeleton below with the correct names of the bones of the body. *(109)*

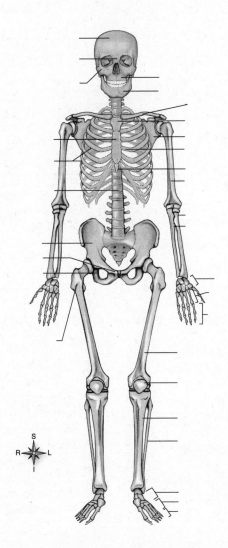

SHORT ANSWER

Directions: Using your own words, answer each question in the space provided.

2. List five functions of the skeletal system. *(108)*

   a. _____

   b. _____

   c. _____

   d. _____

   e. _____

3. List three functions that muscles perform when they contract. *(112)*

   a. _____

   b. _____

   c. _____

4. Discuss neurovascular assessment and include the seven Ps of orthopedic assessment. *(143)* _____

   _____

   _____

   _____

   _____

5. What does "RICE" mean in relation to the treatment for sprains? *(157)* _____

   _____

MULTIPLE CHOICE

Directions: Select the best answer(s) for each of the following questions.

6. The nurse is planning care for several patients on the orthopedic unit. Which patients will need frequent neurovascular checks during the shift? **Select all that apply.** *(137)*
   1. Patient has a long leg cast for fracture sustained in an automobile accident.
   2. Older patient had elective hip replacement surgery secondary to arthritis.
   3. Construction worker sustained a crush injury to the lower leg.
   4. Patient has Volkmann's contracture of the right upper extremity.
   5. Young athlete sustained a dislocated shoulder during a football game.

7. The nurse sees that the patient has a new prescription for alendronate. In addition to medication teaching, which self-care measure is the nurse **most** likely to review with the patient? *(128)*
   1. Fluid intake of at least 2000 mL daily
   2. Postural and breathing exercises
   3. Weight-bearing exercise, such as walking
   4. Application of heat and cold packs for pain

8. The home health nurse is reviewing the medication reconciliation list for a patient who has osteoarthritis. The list includes tramadol, acetaminophen, lisinopril, cortisone, and ibuprofen. Which drug-drug combination is cause for **greatest** concern? *(125)*
   1. Lisinopril and tramadol
   2. Lisinopril and acetaminophen
   3. Lisinopril and cortisone
   4. Lisinopril and ibuprofen

9. What information would the nurse teach about sleep hygiene for a patient who has fibromyalgia? **Select all that apply.** (131)
   1. Take a long, hot bath just before bedtime.
   2. Keep the sleeping environment dark, quiet, and comfortable.
   3. Keep a diary of sleep patterns.
   4. Exercise regularly every day.
   5. Have a protein snack just before going to bed.

10. Which patient needs to be monitored for shock? (145)
    1. Patient reports pain in the muscles, bones, and joints; headaches, altered thought processes, and stiffness.
    2. Patient reports chest pain, especially on inspiration; nurse observes irritability, restlessness, and stupor.
    3. Patient experiences deep, unrelenting, progressive, and poorly localized pain unrelieved by analgesics.
    4. Patient appears anxious, weak, and lethargic; nurse observes hypotension, tachycardia, and diaphoresis.

11. A patient is prescribed colchicine to treat gout. The nurse would assess for which potential medication side effects? (126)
    1. Diarrhea, nausea, and vomiting
    2. Seizures and dysrhythmias
    3. Fluid retention and sodium retention
    4. Hypercalcemia and orthostatic hypotension

12. Which foods should the nurse recommend as good sources of calcium for a 59-year-old woman who is concerned about her risk for osteoporosis? **Select all that apply.** (128)
    1. Milk
    2. Spinach
    3. Potatoes
    4. Sardines
    5. Organ meats

13. The nurse is interviewing a young woman who injured her ankle while playing soccer. Considering the diagnostic testing most likely to be ordered, which question is **most** important to ask? (111)
    1. "Do you have allergies to seafood or iodine?"
    2. "Is there any chance you could be pregnant?"
    3. "Are you currently taking any medications?"
    4. "Do you have a history of radiation exposure?"

14. The nurse is assessing a patient who had a myelogram 3 hours ago. Which patient comment causes the **greatest** concern? (112)
    1. "My head hurts. Could I get an aspirin or a Tylenol tablet?"
    2. "I am thirsty. Would it be okay if I drank a soda or some juice?"
    3. "My foot feels numb and I can't move my toes very well."
    4. "I am not used to lying in bed all day long; I'd like to walk around."

15. The nurse hears in report that the patient has a medical diagnosis of ankylosing spondylitis. What will the nurse include in the focused assessment for this patient? (122)
    1. Perform the 7 Ps of orthopedic assessment.
    2. Assess for back pain and vision changes.
    3. Frequently check for change in mental status.
    4. Check for urinary retention and overflow incontinence.

16. The patient says to the nurse, "I have excruciating pain in my big toe at night." Which assessment question is the nurse **most** likely to ask? (126)
    1. "Have you noticed a change in your bowel movements?"
    2. "How much exercise would you normally get in a week?"
    3. "Do you eat organ meats, yeast, herring, or mackerel?"
    4. "Do you notice jaw tension, excessive fatigue, or anxiety?"

17. The patient is admitted for acute osteomyelitis of the left lower extremity. Which instruction should the nurse give to the unlicensed assistive personnel (UAP)? *(130)*
    1. Use drainage and secretion precautions when caring for the patient.
    2. Assist the patient to ambulate in the hall every 2-3 hours.
    3. Anticipate that movement is more difficult in the morning.
    4. Refresh the patient's ice pack every 2 hours or as needed.

18. The nurse is caring for a patient who had unicompartmental knee surgery. Which interventions will the nurse use in the postoperative period? **Select all that apply.** *(132)*
    1. Encourage deep-breathing and coughing every 2 hours.
    2. Begin with a clear liquid diet and advance to regular as tolerated.
    3. Inspect the skin at the edge of the cast for erythema.
    4. Assess the patient's ability to use an assistive device such as a walker.
    5. Monitor IV fluids and effectiveness of antibiotics.
    6. Administer intraarticular injections of corticosteroids.

19. The patient had a hip arthroplasty and returned from the postanesthesia care unit several hours ago. The patient is now restless and anxious. What is the nurse's **first** action? *(147)*
    1. Decrease anxiety by reassuring the patient that everything is going as expected.
    2. Initiate vital signs every 15 minutes, compare to baseline, and monitor trends.
    3. Look at the urinary output and compare the total to baseline.
    4. Call the patient's family and invite them to spend time at the bedside.

20. A fiberglass cast has been applied to the forearm of a 6-year-old child to treat and stabilize a greenstick fracture. Which teaching point is the **most** important to emphasize with the child? *(146)*
    1. Instructing the child to keep the cast dry
    2. Teaching the child to report pain to the parents
    3. Showing the child how to test capillary refill
    4. Reminding the child to wiggle the fingers

21. The nurse is supervising a nursing student in caring for a patient who had internal fixation for a hip fracture. The nurse would intervene if the student performed which action? *(138)*
    1. Assessed the amount of drainage in the Jackson-Pratt drain
    2. Encouraged coughing and the use of the incentive spirometer
    3. Removed the antiembolism stocking to assess the skin
    4. Placed the patient in high Fowler's position prior to eating

22. The nurse is providing care for a patient who has just had a hip replacement. Which comment from the patient indicates the need for further education? *(134)*
    1. "I need to be on bedrest for the first 72 hours."
    2. "I need to obtain a seat riser for my toilet at home."
    3. "I should never sit with my legs crossed."
    4. "I'll have limitations in hip position for 2-3 months."

23. A nurse is checking on an older neighbor who just fell down. The man cheerfully tells the nurse, "I just tripped on the carpet and took a spill. No harm done!" Based on mechanism of injury, which assessment is the nurse **most** likely to perform if the neighbor will allow it? *(142)*
    1. Head-to-toe to detect occult injury
    2. Palpation and range of motion for wrist injury
    3. Mental status examination for head injury
    4. Environmental assessment for other hazards

24. The patient was in a car accident and reports pain over the pelvic region with difficulty raising legs in a supine position. The nurse notes ecchymosis over the pelvic region. Which laboratory test is the **primary** concern in the immediate phase of care? *(145)*
    1. Hemoglobin and hematocrit
    2. Blood type and Rh
    3. Urinalysis
    4. Stool for occult blood

25. The patient with a cast on the lower extremity reports pain at 7/10. What should the nurse do **first**? *(137)*
    1. Reposition the leg so that elevation is maintained.
    2. Administer pain medication as prescribed.
    3. Report potential compartment syndrome to RN.
    4. Perform the 7 Ps of orthopedic assessment.

26. The nurse hears in report that the patient has Volkmann's contracture of the dominant upper extremity. Which intervention would the nurse plan to use? *(147)*
    1. Frequently assess using the 7 Ps of orthopedic assessment.
    2. Assess the patient's abilities to perform activities of daily living.
    3. Teach the patient to report pain, loss of sensation, or swelling.
    4. Instruct the UAP on proper position and alignment.

27. The nurse is caring for a patient with a long bone fracture. The laboratory reports the following arterial blood gas results. What should the nurse do **first**? *(148)*

pH	7.4
Pa_{CO_2}	40 mm Hg
Pa_{O_2}	95 mm Hg
HCO_3	26 mEq/L
Sa_{O_2}	98%

    1. Assess the patient for signs of fat embolism and respiratory distress.
    2. Report these normal results to the health care provider.
    3. Place the patient in high Fowler's position to ease respirations.
    4. Check the vital signs and continue to monitor the patient.

28. A computer data entry clerk reports paresthesia in the thumb, index finger, and middle finger and pain that increases during the night. The clerk has an appointment with a health care provider next week. In the meantime, what self-care measure would the nurse advise? *(161)*
    1. Use warm packs and sleep with hands on a pillow.
    2. Frequently change position and stretch hands while working.
    3. Use a mild analgesic such as ibuprofen or aspirin.
    4. Wrap the wrist snugly with an elastic bandage.

29. The patient who had a laminectomy reports abdominal discomfort with a gaseous, bloated feeling and mild nausea. What should the nurse do **first**? *(163)*
    1. Offer clear liquids.
    2. Encourage ambulation.
    3. Listen for bowel sounds.
    4. Administer an antiemetic.

30. The patient reports long bone pain that increases with weight bearing. The health care provider tells the nurse that the patient has an elevated serum alkaline phosphatase. The nurse prepares to give emotional support because the provider must tell the patient that additional diagnostic testing is needed to rule out which condition? *(163)*
    1. Phantom limb pain
    2. Compartment syndrome
    3. Fibromyalgia
    4. Osteogenic sarcoma

CRITICAL THINKING ACTIVITIES

Activity 1

31. Discuss factors that contribute to osteoporosis and the nurse's role in helping patients prevent bone loss and fractures. *(127-129)*

_____

_____

_____

_____

_____

Activity 2

32. A 32-year-old woman has been told that she might have fibromyalgia syndrome; however, the health care provider tells her that this is just a possibility and that additional diagnostic testing would be needed. The patient is angry at first and then she begins to cry and confides in the nurse, "I am just so frustrated with these doctors and I just want to be able to live a normal life." Discuss fibromyalgia syndrome from the patient's point of view. *(130, 131)*

_____

_____

_____

_____

_____

Activity 3

33. The home health nurse is visiting a thin, older woman who lives alone. The three-story house is a little cluttered with old belongings. Her bedroom and bathroom are on the second floor. The rugs are worn and the hallways are poorly lit. The woman cheerfully reports that she has a cane, a walker, and eyeglasses, but frequently misplaces "all of the 'old person' stuff." The woman has a small friendly dog; he jumps at her legs and she frequently bends down to pet him. Discuss the potential for hip fracture for this woman. *(136)*

_____

_____

_____

_____

_____

Care of the Patient With a Gastrointestinal Disorder

Answer Key: Textbook page references are provided as a guide for answering these questions. A complete Answer Key is provided in your Additional Learning Resources on Evolve.

FIGURE LABELING

1. Directions: Label the digestive organs. *(172)*

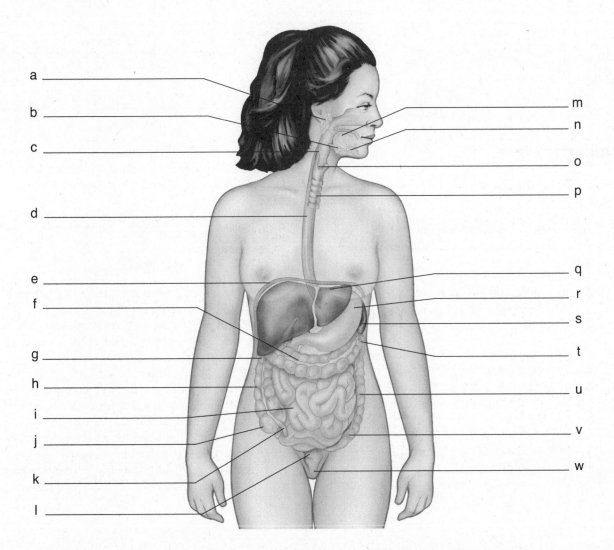

a _____

b _____

c _____

d _____

e _____

f _____

g _____

h _____

i _____

j _____

k _____

l _____

m _____

n _____

o _____

p _____

q _____

r _____

s _____

t _____

u _____

v _____

w _____

SHORT ANSWER

Directions: Using your own words, answer each question in the space provided.

2. List three functions of saliva. *(173)*

   a. _____

   b. _____

   c. _____

3. List four major functions of the large intestine. *(174)*

   a. _____

   b. _____

   c. _____

   d. _____

4. The liver is a complex organ that has many functions; name four or five of these functions. *(175)*

   _____

   _____

   _____

   _____

MULTIPLE CHOICE

Directions: Select the best answer(s) for each of the following questions.

5. According to research, removal or disease of the appendix could theoretically affect which function? *(174)*
   1. Immunologic response
   2. Red blood cell production
   3. Fluid and electrolyte balance
   4. Vitamin B$_{12}$ production

6. The large intestine is the site of bacterial action that produces vitamin K. Potentially, loss of the large colon or disruption of this bacterial action could disrupt which body function? *(175)*
   1. Color vision
   2. Bone formation
   3. Intestinal absorption
   4. Blood clotting

7. What is the **most** important postprocedure instruction to give to a patient who has had an upper gastrointestinal study with barium? *(178)*
   1. Watch for and report bleeding.
   2. Monitor temperature.
   3. Increase fluid intake.
   4. Eat a low-residue diet.

8. The nurse is planning care for several patients who will be undergoing diagnostic testing for disorders of the gastrointestinal system. Which patient is going to require the **most** time for postprocedural care? *(177)*
   1. Patient must undergo capsule endoscopy to confirm diagnosis of celiac disease.
   2. Patient needs an esophagogastroduodenoscopy for evaluation of an ulcer.
   3. Patient is scheduled for a barium swallow to evaluate extent of hiatal hernia.
   4. Patient is tested for *H. pylori*: breath, serum antibody test, and fecal assay antigen.

9. The patient reports a substernal burning sensation that radiates into the neck and jaw. He says, "I think it's heartburn." The nurse decides to check vital signs and conduct further assessments of the pain. What is the **best** rationale for the nurse's decision? *(183)*
   1. Pain assessment is performed before and after offering medication or nonpharmacologic interventions.
   2. Report to the health care provider should include vital signs and a description of the signs/symptoms.
   3. Heartburn can lead to more serious conditions, such as hemorrhage, sepsis, or cancer.
   4. The subjective sensations mimic angina and a potential cardiac condition should not be overlooked.

10. Which patient situation **most** strongly indicates the need for further investigation as a potential public health problem? *(197)*
    1. Patient develops symptoms of acute gastritis after excessive drinking at a local bar.
    2. Patient has bloody diarrhea after eating a grilled hamburger that was served at a fundraiser.
    3. Patient has a burning sensation and regurgitation after eating spicy food at an ethnic restaurant.
    4. Patient has abdominal bloating and muscle aches after eating pastry at a local bakery.

11. What are the common causes of fecal incontinence? **Select all that apply.** *(221)*
    1. Normal changes of aging
    2. Injury during anal intercourse
    3. Surgical trauma to anal sphincter
    4. Injury during childbirth
    5. Spinal cord lesions
    6. Voluntary inhibition of defecation

12. When planning care for a patient with a motor paralysis, which intervention is the **most** important as a long-term solution for the patient's defecation? *(221)*
    1. Teach the family and patient the logroll to clean fecal incontinence.
    2. Include the patient and family in planning a bowel training program.
    3. Contact social services to find funds for incontinence pads and briefs.
    4. Arrange for home health services for assistance with hygiene and toileting.

13. Which patient is the **best** candidate for a bowel training program that will incorporate biofeedback? *(221)*
    1. Patient has structural damage to the rectum secondary to a fistula.
    2. Patient has a motility disorder but is alert and motivated.
    3. Patient is ambulatory but has mild dementia and forgetfulness.
    4. Patient is passing liquid stool secondary to a fecal impaction.

14. The patient is practicing a bowel training program. Which food will the nurse encourage the patient to eat? *(221)*
    1. Lean chicken meat
    2. Low-fat milk
    3. Whole-grain cereal
    4. Red meat

15. A patient is being treated with sucralfate for gastroesophageal reflux disease. Which teaching point would the nurse emphasize? *(191)*
    1. Oral anticoagulants, theophylline, and propranolol may require dosage reductions.
    2. Coating action may interfere with the absorption of other drugs—separate by 2 hours.
    3. Contraindicated during pregnancy; women of childbearing age must use reliable contraception.
    4. Avoid driving or other hazardous activities until accustomed to sedating effects.

16. A patient had a partial gastrectomy. Because this surgery creates an increased risk for pernicious anemia, which teaching point is important to emphasize? *(196)*
    1. Blood serum vitamin B_{12} level should be measured every 1 to 2 years.
    2. Hemoglobin and hematocrit should be measured every 1 to 2 months.
    3. Injections of iron dextran are given because of intestinal ulceration.
    4. Increase fresh fruits and vegetables and decrease intake of fat and red meat.

17. The risk of cancer of the stomach is associated with which factors? **Select all that apply.** *(194)*
    1. Hyperkalemia
    2. Hypochlorhydria
    3. Chronic atrophic gastritis
    4. Diet high in smoked and preserved foods
    5. Gastric ulcers
    6. Diet low in fresh fruits and whole grains

18. When caring for a patient diagnosed with Crohn's disease, what signs and symptoms does the nurse expect to observe? **Select all that apply.** (206)
    1. Nausea and vomiting
    2. Diarrhea and abdominal pain
    3. Weight gain and lactose intolerance
    4. Weight loss and malnutrition
    5. Fatigue and fever

19. The nurse is providing care to a patient suspected of having acute appendicitis. Which interventions may be included in the care? **Select all that apply.** (208)
    1. Apply heating pad to the abdomen.
    2. Maintain bedrest and nothing by mouth (NPO).
    3. Administer antacids as needed to decrease gastric acidity.
    4. Monitor vital signs including temperature.
    5. Administer antibiotics as prescribed.
    6. Administer enemas until clear.

20. The patient had an esophagogastroduodenoscopy several hours ago and now reports abdominal pain and tenderness. What should the nurse do **first**? (177)
    1. Auscultate for bowel sounds.
    2. Administer pain medication.
    3. Assess the abdominal pain.
    4. Check for melena.

21. The patient had capsule endoscopy. Which discharge instruction should the nurse give to the patient? (177)
    1. The capsule will pass with bowel movement in 2-3 days; no need to retrieve.
    2. Use gloves and examine stool for several days to retrieve pill camera device.
    3. Use a mild laxative and increase liquids to facilitate expulsion of pill camera.
    4. Small amounts of light red blood and thick mucus in the stool are expected.

22. The nurse inserts a nasogastric tube so a patient can undergo the Bernstein test to determine the cause of esophageal pain. Which outcome is considered a positive test result? (177)
    1. Administering nitrates relieves pain.
    2. Taking an antacid has no effect on pain.
    3. Decompressing the stomach relieves pain.
    4. Instilling hydrochloric acid causes pain.

23. The patient needs to have a series of tests of the gastrointestinal system. Which test must be scheduled last? (179)
    1. Barium studies
    2. Stool sample for ova and parasites
    3. Colonoscopy
    4. Flat plate of the abdomen

24. The nursing student reports seeing a pearly, bluish-white "milk-curd" on the mucous membranes of the older patient's mouth. The nurse would intervene if the student performs which action? (180)
    1. Checks for angular cheilitis at the corner of the mouth
    2. Removes the plaques with a soft toothbrush
    3. Observes the quantity and type of food consumed
    4. Offers the patient unsweetened yogurt

25. The nurse is talking to a neighbor who says that she has had a sore on her lip for about 3 weeks. What advice should the nurse give? (181)
    1. Use lipstick or lip balm that has a sunscreen.
    2. Advise rinsing the mouth with diluted hydrogen peroxide.
    3. Consult the health care provider because of the duration of the sore.
    4. Increase intake of fresh fruits and vegetables for vitamin content.

26. The health care provider has recommended a conservative approach to manage the patient's gastroesophageal reflux disease. What would be included in the nurse's instructions to support the provider's recommendation? (183)
    1. Give the patient a brochure about Nissen fundoplication.
    2. Suggest methods for elevating the head of the bed at home.
    3. Teach the signs and symptoms of Barrett's esophagus.
    4. Give the patient a reminder card for endoscopy and biopsy.

27. The nurse is caring for a patient who was admitted for peptic ulcer disease. Which abnormal finding is the **greatest** concern? *(188)*
    1. Fecal assay antigen test is positive for *H. pylori*.
    2. Stool for occult blood is positive.
    3. White blood cell count is elevated.
    4. Pain is present during the hydrochloric acid test.

28. The patient who had surgery for a peptic ulcer several weeks ago reports experiencing an episode of diaphoresis, nausea, vomiting, epigastric pain, explosive diarrhea, and dyspepsia. Which question is **most** relevant to the symptoms and the surgical history? *(196)*
    1. "Can you describe the pain? Where was it and how long did it last?"
    2. "Did you eat before the symptoms? And if so, what did you eat?"
    3. "Have you been taking your medications according to instructions?"
    4. "Did you ever experience these symptoms before the surgery?"

29. The patient is admitted for hemorrhagic colitis caused by the *E. coli* pathogen. Which order would the nurse question? *(197)*
    1. Encourage oral fluids as tolerated
    2. Dextrose 5% in normal saline at 150 mL/ hour
    3. Loperamide 2 mg after unformed stool
    4. Initiate contact isolation

30. The older adult patient has been put into contact isolation because of watery diarrhea. Laboratory results are pending, but the *C. difficile* pathogen is suspected. What instruction should the nurse give to the unlicensed assistive personnel? *(197)*
    1. Cluster care and limit the amount of time spent in the room.
    2. Use diluted bleach solution to clean the toilet bowl after each use.
    3. Wear a mask during patient care and discard upon exiting the room.
    4. Use soap and water to wash hands, rather than the antiseptic hand rub.

31. The nurse is assisting a patient who is newly diagnosed with celiac disease. Which lunch tray would be the **best** choice? *(199)*
    1. Whole-grain pasta with marinara and a green salad
    2. Chicken breast sandwich on rye bread and an apple
    3. Chicken noodle soup and crackers with fruit salad
    4. Stir-fry vegetables with rice and orange slices

32. The patient confides in the nurse that she feels angry because the health care provider has hinted that irritable bowel syndrome (IBS) might be the problem but offers no definitive medical diagnosis. What is the **most** therapeutic response? *(200)*
    1. "IBS is hard to diagnose. It is more a process of excluding other disorders."
    2. "I'll ask the health care provider to talk to you about your concerns."
    3. "You seem really frustrated. What has the provider told you so far?"
    4. "I can get some literature about IBS; maybe additional information will help."

33. The patient is admitted for an exacerbation of ulcerative colitis and the nurse hears in report that the patient had 20 liquid stools within the past 24 hours. Which laboratory result is the **most** important to follow up on? *(202)*
    1. Electrolyte levels
    2. Liver function studies
    3. Hemoglobin and hematocrit
    4. Fecal occult blood

34. The nurse enters the room of a young woman and sees that she is crying. The patient states, "The doctor told me I need surgery and an ileostomy. I'll be pooping into a bag! I'm leaving the hospital right now!" What should the nurse do **first**? *(218)*
    1. Obtain a leaving Against Medical Advice form and contact the provider.
    2. Sit with the patient and help her verbalize her fears and concerns.
    3. Arrange for the patient to meet another person who has an ostomy.
    4. Contact the enterostomal therapist to talk with the patient.

35. Which medical diagnosis requires that the nurse be extra vigilant for concurrent urinary tract infections? *(206)*
    1. Crohn's disease
    2. Appendicitis
    3. Ulcerative colitis
    4. Peptic ulcer disease

36. A parent says, "I think my son has an appendicitis. He won't eat and he says he has pain just to the right of his belly button." If the nurse places the child on an examination table, which position is the child **most** likely to assume if the mother is correct about appendicitis? *(208)*
    1. Prone with head supported by forearm
    2. Supine with arms and legs extended
    3. Sits upright, with chest extended
    4. Side-lying with knees flexed

37. The patient is admitted for acute diverticulitis. The nurse would intervene if a nursing student performed which action? *(209)*
    1. Advises to avoid heavy lifting
    2. Assists with a meal tray
    3. Assesses bowel sounds
    4. Checks the white blood cell count

38. A patient sustained blunt trauma to the abdomen. Several hours after being admitted for observation, the patient reports severe abdominal pain with exquisite tenderness to light palpation. What should the nurse do **first**? *(211)*
    1. Take vital signs and perform additional assessment of the abdomen.
    2. Place the patient in a semi-Fowler's position to localize purulent drainage.
    3. Call the health care provider and report possible peritonitis.
    4. Administer an as-needed pain medication and reevaluate pain in 30 minutes.

39. The nurse is caring for a patient who had a right hemicolectomy for colorectal cancer. Which postoperative interventions will the nurse use in the care of this patient? **Select all that apply.** *(218)*
    1. Monitor vital signs, pain level, and return of bowel sounds.
    2. Check dressings for drainage and bleeding and change as ordered.
    3. Discontinue the urinary catheter when the patient is discharged.
    4. Encourage the patient to cough, deep-breathe, and turn.
    5. Maintain bedrest while the nasogastric tube is on suction.
    6. Keep accurate intake and output records to monitor fluid balance.

40. An obese male truck driver comes to the clinic and reports intense rectal itching. The health care provider determines that the patient has hemorrhoids. What nonsurgical approach can the nurse teach the patient to help manage the condition? *(219)*
    1. Suggest a low-fiber diet.
    2. Advise the use of a hydrocortisone cream.
    3. Increase fluid intake.
    4. Recommend rubber-band ligation.

41. What is considered an **early** sign of mechanical obstruction of the intestines? *(214)*
    1. Loud, frequent, high-pitched bowel sounds
    2. Intermittent periods of decreased or absent bowel sounds
    3. Decreased blood pressure with tachycardia
    4. Abdominal distention and vomiting

42. Which sign/symptom should be investigated as an **early** warning of colorectal cancer? *(216)*
    1. Abdominal distention
    2. Rectal bleeding
    3. Nausea
    4. Weight loss

CRITICAL THINKING ACTIVITIES

Activity 1

43. The patient reports a burning sensation in the mid-epigastric area after eating, and occasionally experiences a feeling of warm fluid moving up the throat with a sour taste in the mouth. The health care provider makes the medical diagnosis of gastroesophageal reflux disease and suggests trying lifestyle modifications. Discuss the dietary interventions and lifestyle modifications that the nurse will reinforce. *(184)*

_____

_____

_____

_____

_____

_____

Activity 2

44. A 24-year-old male patient presents with weakness, loss of appetite, abdominal pain and cramps, intermittent low-grade fever, sleeplessness caused by diarrhea, and stress. The health care provider recommends diagnostic colonoscopy and laboratory testing and identifies the medical diagnosis of Crohn's disease and sulfasalazine is prescribed. The dietitian is consulted and provides extensive teaching about dietary strategies to manage the disease process. Discuss Crohn's disease from the patient's point of view. *(206, 207)*

_____

_____

_____

_____

_____

_____

Activity 3

45. The nurse has taken a new job at a long-term care center. With regards to the gastrointestinal system, what are some of the lifespan considerations that the nurse is likely to observe while caring for this group of older adults? *(213)*

_____

_____

_____

_____

_____

Activity 4

46. The nurse is providing care to a patient suspected of having an intestinal obstruction. *(213-215)*

    a.   When performing an assessment on the patient, what objective data should be included?

          _____

          _____

    b.   What diagnostic tests may be performed to confirm the presence of an intestinal obstruction?

          _____

          _____

    c.   What are the goals of treatment for an intestinal obstruction? _____

          _____

          _____

    d.   Compare mechanical and nonmechanical intestinal obstruction. _____

          _____

          _____

Care of the Patient With a Gallbladder, Liver, Biliary Tract, or Exocrine Pancreatic Disorder

Answer Key: Textbook page references are provided as a guide for answering these questions. A complete Answer Key is provided in your Additional Learning Resources on Evolve.

SHORT ANSWER

Directions: Using your own words, answer each question in the space provided.

1. Identify at least five modifiable risk factors for pancreatic cancer. *(250)* _____

_____

_____

_____

_____

MULTIPLE CHOICE

Directions: Select the best answer(s) for each of the following questions.

2. The nurse hears in report that the patient has a total bilirubin of 2.8 mg/dL. What would the nurse expect to observe during the morning assessment? *(225)*
   1. Jaundice of the sclera and mucous membranes
   2. Pallor of the palms of hands and soles of feet
   3. Cyanosis of the lips with minor exertion
   4. Cherry red discoloration of the face and chest

3. The home health nurse sees that the patient's albumin level is 3.4 g/dL. Based on this information, which assessment is the nurse **most** likely to perform? *(226)*
   1. Frequency and type of exercise and physical activity
   2. Dietary preferences and typical intake for 24-hour period
   3. Frequency of using tobacco or illicit substances
   4. Occupational or other environmental exposure to toxins.

4. The nurse is responsible for the postprocedural care of several patients who had diagnostic testing. The unlicensed assistive personnel (UAP) reports that one of the patients is having shortness of breath; rapid, shallow breathing; and a rapid pulse. Which patient is **most** likely to develop these signs/symptoms as a postprocedural complication? *(228)*
   1. Patient had a radioisotope scan of the liver.
   2. Patient had ultrasonography of the pancreas.
   3. Patient had computed tomography of the abdomen.
   4. Patient had a needle biopsy of the liver.

5. The nurse is caring for an older patient who becomes confused and combative under stressful situations or during changes in routine. The health care provider has ordered several diagnostic tests. The nurse is **most** likely to contact the provider before scheduling which test? *(230)*
   1. 2-hour spot urine for urine amylase
   2. Serum ammonia test
   3. Endoscopic retrograde cholangiopancreatography
   4. Total protein and serum albumin

6. The patient has a damaged liver and is therefore unable to correctly metabolize protein. Loss of this function results in portal hypertension, hypoalbuminemia, and hyperaldosteronism. Based on the nurse's knowledge of pathophysiology, what would the nurse expect to observe when assessing the patient? *(232)*
   1. Flatulence
   2. Ascites
   3. Asterixis
   4. Cachexia

7. What are **early** signs/symptoms of cirrhosis of the liver? *(232)*
   1. Esophageal varices
   2. Spider angiomas
   3. Ascites
   4. Flulike symptoms

8. The home health nurse is visiting a patient who has cirrhosis of the liver. Which patient behavior is cause for **greatest** concern? *(236)*
   1. Patient nicked his face several times while using a razor blade for shaving.
   2. Patient bumped his head on the doorway and now seems mildly confused.
   3. Patient noticed bleeding from the gums after brushing teeth and flossing.
   4. Patient has ecchymotic spots on his forearms and back of the hands.

9. The health care provider may prescribe a protein-restricted diet for which patient? *(228)*
   1. Patient is recovering from acute hepatic encephalopathy.
   2. Patient is in the early stage of cirrhosis of the liver.
   3. Patient is being treated conservatively for cholecystitis.
   4. Patient is recovering from hepatitis A, contracted 3 months ago.

10. Which people should be advised to get the hepatitis B vaccine (HBV)? **Select all that apply.** *(240)*
    1. Nurse who works in the emergency department
    2. Person who injects illicit substances
    3. Groundskeeper who works at an inner city park
    4. Newborn who is having a 2-month well-baby examination
    5. Older resident who lives in a long-term care facility
    6. Military person who is stationed in a developing country

11. The nurse hears in report that the patient has hepatic encephalopathy and is receiving lactulose. What will the nurse observe if the medication therapy is successful? *(235)*
    1. Improved mental status
    2. Decreased ascites
    3. Improved appetite
    4. Decreased jaundice

12. What instructions should be given to the UAP about the care of a patient with viral hepatitis? **Select all that apply.** *(239)*
    1. Perform scrupulous hand hygiene.
    2. Wear gown and gloves when handling excreta.
    3. Exercise caution when putting needles in the sharps box.
    4. Wear a mask if bedside care is extensive or prolonged.
    5. Organize care to reduce time and exposure to the patient.

13. The patient had a laparoscopic cholecystectomy yesterday and is schedule to be discharged today. Which assessment finding would delay the discharge? *(246)*
    1. Patient reports mild shoulder pain.
    2. Patient reports pain when T-tube is clamped.
    3. Patient notices bile leakage from the puncture site.
    4. Patient eats but his appetite is not at baseline.

14. The nurse is providing teaching to a patient scheduled to undergo a needle biopsy of the liver. During the examination, what will the patient be told to do? *(227)*
    1. Deeply inhale and hold breath until instructed to exhale.
    2. Cough forcefully as the needle is withdrawn.
    3. Inhale and exhale slowly and evenly as the needle is inserted.
    4. Exhale and hold breath as the needle is inserted.

15. A T-tube was inserted during a cholecystectomy. What does the nurse expect to observe when assessing the patient? *(247)*
    1. Greenish-yellow drainage from the tube
    2. Localized inflammation around the tube site
    3. Significant postoperative pain until the tube is removed
    4. Moderate amount of light-red bleeding from the tube

16. After a laparoscopic cholecystectomy, the patient reports shoulder pain. What should the nurse do? *(246)*
    1. Perform gentle range-of-motion exercises to reduce shoulder discomfort.
    2. Assist the patient to ambulate to clear the residual carbon dioxide.
    3. Explain that the pain is an expected side effect of anesthesia.
    4. Reassure that the pain is expected and give an analgesic as prescribed.

17. When caring for a patient with acute pancreatitis, which laboratory finding is the **best** indicator of the disorder? *(248)*
    1. Low albumin
    2. Elevated lipase
    3. Increased blood glucose
    4. Elevated amylase

18. Which behavior places a person at **greatest** risk to contract hepatitis E? *(239)*
    1. Eating raw shellfish or drinking water in Mexico
    2. Engaging in unprotected anal and vaginal sex
    3. Sharing and reusing needles for illicit drug injection
    4. Getting tattooed with nonsterile equipment

19. The nurse hears in report that the patient had lithotripsy for gallstones. Which postprocedural assessment is the nurse most likely to perform? *(244-245)*
    1. Assess for drainage at the incision site
    2. Assess level of pain and discomfort
    3. Assess for nausea and amount of emesis
    4. Assess ability to do activities of daily living

20. A young woman who is pregnant is having symptoms of cholecystitis and the health care provider has informed her that diagnostic testing is required. Which educational brochure will the nurse prepare for this patient? *(227)*
    1. "What You Need to Know About Ultrasonography of the Gallbladder"
    2. "Frequently Asked Questions About Oral Cholecystography"
    3. "Intravenous Cholangiography: A Patient's Guide for Decision-making"
    4. "Computed Tomography of the Abdomen as a Diagnostic Tool"

21. The patient had a hepatobiliary iminodiacetic acid (HIDA) scan. What instructions should the nurse give to the UAP who is assisting the patient with hygiene? *(227)*
    1. Immediately flush all urine and stool.
    2. Wear your personal dosimeter at all times.
    3. Give care as usual; there are no special considerations.
    4. Watch for and report any bleeding at the puncture site.

22. The nurse hears in report that several patients are scheduled for diagnostic testing. The nurse must plan to frequently take vital signs (every 15 minutes x 2, then every 30 minutes x 4 , and then every hour x 4) after which test? *(228)*
    1. Serum ammonia test
    2. Needle liver biopsy
    3. Oral cholecystography
    4. Radioisotope liver scan

23. The nurse is instructing the UAP about assisting several patients with morning hygiene. Which patient needs to use a soft toothbrush with very gentle brushing action? *(236)*
    1. Recently diagnosed with hepatitis A
    2. Surgery pending for cholelithiasis
    3. In later stage of cirrhosis of the liver
    4. Nothing by mouth for acute pancreatitis

24. A first-semester nursing student tells the nurse that she would like to teach and coach coughing and deep-breathing to several patients. Which patients would be **best** for the nurse to recommend to the student? **Select all that apply.** *(234)*
    1. Scheduled to have a cholecystectomy in 2 days
    2. Looks forward to having a liver transplant from a living donor
    3. Has cirrhosis of the liver and esophageal varices
    4. Prescribed several weeks of bedrest for chronic hepatitis
    5. Is on bedrest for acute pancreatitis with severe pain

25. The patient has symptoms of hepatic encephalopathy and the health care provider wants to be called about laboratory results. Which laboratory result should the nurse seek out to validate the suspected condition? *(228)*
    1. Serum bilirubin
    2. Serum albumin
    3. Ammonia level
    4. Blood glucose

26. The health care provider orders an intramuscular immune serum globulin for a hospital employee who was exposed to hepatitis A. A dosage of 0.2 mL/kg of body weight is ordered. The employee weighs 155 lbs. How many mL should the nurse draw up? _____ mL *(240)*

27. A patient with acute pancreatitis is refusing to have a nasogastric tube inserted and wants to leave the hospital. What can the nurse say to help the patient to accept the therapy? *(249)*
    1. "I can give you pain medication before or after the procedure."
    2. "Let me call the health care provider so he can explain the therapy."
    3. "The tube will be inserted by our most experienced nurse, so don't worry."
    4. "The tube will decrease the nausea, vomiting, pain, and abdominal distention."

CRITICAL THINKING ACTIVITIES

Activity 1

28. A 34-year-old patient with a history of end-stage liver disease related to chronic hepatitis has been added to the waiting list to receive a liver transplant. During his preoperative education classes, he voices many questions and concerns. *(241)*

    a. What are the primary risks associated with the planned transplant? _____

        _____

    b. For which postoperative complications will the patient be at risk?_____

        _____

        _____

    c. How will the risk of organ rejection be handled?_____

        _____

        _____

        _____

    d. Discuss the appropriate postoperative nursing care._____

        _____

        _____

        _____

Activity 2

29. A 49-year-old patient comes to the emergency department for right upper-quadrant pain. She reports that the pain began a few hours after eating French fries, a hamburger, and an ice cream sundae at a local fast-food restaurant. Upon assessment, the abdomen is distended. The patient also has nausea and vomiting. *(243, 244)*

    a. What does the nurse expect the patient to be diagnosed with? _____

    b. What are some other signs and symptoms that may develop? _____

        _____

    c. What diagnostic examinations may be used to help diagnose this patient? _____

        _____

        _____

        _____

Activity 3

30. a. Based on knowledge of the etiology and clinical course of pancreatic cancer, discuss some of the psychological challenges that a patient could face. *(250, 251)*

   _____

   _____

   _____

   _____

   b. What can the nurse do to assist the patient with these psychological challenges? *(250, 251)* _____

   _____

   _____

   _____

   _____

Care of the Patient With a Blood or Lymphatic Disorder

Answer Key: Textbook page references are provided as a guide for answering these questions. A complete Answer Key is provided in your Additional Learning Resources on Evolve.

SHORT ANSWER

Directions: Using your own words, answer each question in the space provided.

1. What are the three main functions of blood? *(256)* _____

   _____

   _____

   _____

2. What are three functions of the lymphatic system? *(260)* _____

   _____

   _____

3. What are two main functions of the lymph glands? *(261)* _____

   _____

4. What are five functions of the spleen? *(261)* _____

   _____

   _____

   _____

   _____

TABLE ACTIVITY

5. Directions: Complete the table below with the normal values for selected blood tests. *(256)*

Blood Test	Normal Values		
Red blood cells (RBCs)	Males:		Females:
Hemoglobin	Males:		Females:
Hematocrit	Males:		Females:
Platelet count			
White blood cells (WBC) actual cell count			
Prothrombin time (PT)			
International Normalized Ratio (INR)			
Partial thromboplastin time (PTT)			

MULTIPLE CHOICE

Directions: Select the best answer(s) for each of the following questions.

6. There was a major catastrophe in the city and health care facilities are being overwhelmed with trauma victims. Based on the concept of universal recipient, which patient theoretically has the **best** chance of getting a unit of blood if there is a shortage in the blood banks? *(259)*
   1. Has blood type O and is Rh negative
   2. Has blood type A and is Rh positive
   3. Has blood type B and is Rh negative
   4. Has blood type AB and is Rh positive

7. During physical assessment, the nurse detects swelling in the cervical lymph nodes and the patient's skin feels hot to the touch. Which question is the nurse **most** likely to ask to follow up on the assessment findings? *(261)*
   1. "Do you have a personal or family history of cancer?"
   2. "Have you ever been told that you were anemic?"
   3. "Have you been exposed to any infectious disorders?"
   4. "Do you take any anticoagulant medications?"

8. Which patient has the **greatest** risk for developing a complication related to the penetration of underlying structures during a bone marrow biopsy or aspiration? *(262)*
   1. An older patient had a bone marrow biopsy from the posterior iliac crest.
   2. A very thin patient had a bone marrow aspiration from the sternum.
   3. A child had a bone marrow aspiration from the posterior iliac crest.
   4. An obese patient had a bone marrow aspiration from the tibia.

9. Which objective finding indicates that the healthy adult's body is compensating for a blood loss of less than 750 mL? *(263)*
   1. Urine output is scant.
   2. Blood pressure is low.
   3. Has slight increase in pulse.
   4. Is stuporous and confused.

10. The patient is admitted for an exacerbation of polycythemia vera. Which patient report is cause for **greatest** concern? *(273)*
    1. Reports pain in lower leg with redness and swelling
    2. Has generalized pruritus after taking a hot shower
    3. Reports fullness and satiety after eating a small salad
    4. Has burning sensation of the hands and feet

11. Which lunch tray is the **best** choice for providing nutrients needed for erythropoiesis? *(270)*
    1. Fried egg, potato and cheese burrito, low-fat milk, and an apple
    2. Chicken breast sandwich with fries, low-fat milk with vanilla yogurt
    3. Fresh fruit salad with whole-grain roll and strawberry smoothie
    4. Spinach salad with nuts and strawberries and tuna on whole-grain bread

12. The nurse is caring for a young patient who is usually very healthy, but has vomiting and diarrhea secondary to food poisoning. What would be an expected laboratory result for this patient? *(256)*
    1. Elevated hemoglobin and hematocrit
    2. Normal hemoglobin and hematocrit
    3. Low platelet count
    4. Increased prothrombin time

13. The health care provider tells the nurse that the laboratory results show that the patient has bandemia. The nurse will plan to be extra vigilant for which condition? *(258)*
    1. Venous thrombosis
    2. Thrombocytopenia
    3. Sepsis or septic shock
    4. Allergic response

14. Which patient is **most** likely to require testing for anti-D antibodies and/or an injection of Rh immunoglobulin? *(260)*
    1. An Rh-positive mother who is at 28 weeks gestation
    2. Any woman who has an ectopic pregnancy
    3. An Rh-negative mother who had a miscarriage
    4. An Rh-positive mother impregnated by an Rh-negative father

15. When caring for patients who are Jehovah's Witnesses, which information applies for use of blood products? *(264)*
    1. Some Jehovah's Witnesses may permit the use of certain blood volume expanders.
    2. It is not legal for this patient to refuse transfusions if the bleeding is truly life-threatening.
    3. Some Jehovah's Witnesses may consent to homologous blood transfusions.
    4. Jehovah's Witnesses believe that children are allowed to have blood in an emergency.

16. A patient with anemia has difficulty with activities because of tissue hypoxia. Which task can be delegated to the UAP? *(264)*
    1. Ask the patient how far he is able to ambulate and evaluate his abilities.
    2. Apply oxygen per nasal cannula if the patient reports shortness of breath.
    3. Explain the patient's limitations to visitors and encourage short visits.
    4. Assist the patient with self-care activities such as hygiene and toileting.

17. The nurse is caring for a trauma patient who must be observed for signs and symptoms of occult bleeding and injury. Which sign/symptom is an **early** manifestation of hypovolemic shock? *(264)*
    1. Orthostatic blood pressure
    2. Decreased red blood cell count
    3. Restlessness
    4. Decreased urine output

18. The patient had major abdominal surgery yesterday. He reported abdominal pain, and the nurse gave him an opioid pain medication as directed; 2 hours later, he reports that the pain is worse. What should the nurse do **first**? *(265)*
    1. Check the medication administration record for other pain or adjunctive medications.
    2. Explain to the patient that pain medication can only be given as prescribed every 4-6 hours.
    3. Reassess the abdomen and ask the patient to describe the pain to the best of his ability.
    4. Call the health care provider and obtain an order for laboratory studies or x-ray studies.

19. The nurse is caring for a postoperative patient who is demonstrating early symptoms of hypovolemic shock. The nurse is awaiting a return call from the health care provider. Which task can be delegated to the UAP? *(265)*
    1. Take and report the blood pressure, pulse, and respirations every 15 minutes.
    2. Reinforce the dressings for saturation of blood or drainage.
    3. Apply oxygen and monitor the pulse oximetry readings every 5 minutes.
    4. Place the patient in a supine position and monitor respiratory effort.

20. The health care provider has recommended that the patient with sickle cell disease have a splenectomy. Which medication is likely to be discontinued for several days prior to the surgery? *(268)*
    1. Folic acid supplement
    2. Hydroxyurea
    3. Blood thinner
    4. Antibiotic

21. The nurse is caring for a patient experiencing an initial sickle cell crisis. What is the **primary** sign/symptom that the nurse should expect during the crisis? *(271)*
    1. Jaundice
    2. Fever
    3. Fatigue
    4. Pain

22. What health promotion points should be emphasized for patients who have sickle cell disease? **Select all that apply.** *(272)*
    1. Avoid high altitudes
    2. Drink large amounts of iced fluids
    3. Stay current with vaccinations
    4. Maintain very cold room temperatures
    5. Stop smoking and alcohol consumption
    6. Maintain vigorous exercise routine

23. The patient is diagnosed with primary polycythemia. Which assessments are the **most** important? *(273)*
    1. Palpating for abdominal distention and checking bowel movements
    2. Checking for pain, warmth, swelling, redness, and pulses in arms or legs
    3. Monitoring temperature and watching for other signs of infection
    4. Frequently assessing for fatigue and activity intolerance

24. The laboratory calls to inform the nurse that the patient has a white cell count of $1000/mm^3$ with a differential neutrophil count of less than $200/mm^3$. Which action is the **most** important for the nurse to initiate while waiting for the health care provider to respond to the phone message? *(275)*
    1. Review current medication list.
    2. Start neutropenic precautions.
    3. Check for signs/symptoms of infection.
    4. Teach the importance of hand hygiene. .

25. A 6-year-old child is hospitalized for treatment of acute lymphocytic leukemia. Which activity would the nurse suggest to the child and parents? *(275, 276)*
    1. Drawing pictures that accompany storytelling
    2. Playing with and petting the pet therapy dog
    3. Walking in the garden courtyard
    4. Attending a party in the pediatric play area

26. The nurse is examining the patient and notices several areas of ecchymoses and petechiae. Which question(s) will the nurse ask to follow up on this observation? **Select all that apply.** *(278)*
    1. "What do you think is causing these bruises?"
    2. "Do you notice any bleeding when you brush your teeth?"
    3. "Have you had frequent nosebleeds?"
    4. "Are your stools a black or very dark red color?"
    5. "Are you using a hydrocortisone cream on these areas?"
    6. "How much dietary fiber do you consume per day?"

27. The patient has a very low platelet count. Which instruction will the nurse give to the UAP about the care of this patient? *(278)*
    1. Always wear a mask to prevent spreading respiratory droplets.
    2. Handle the patient very gently to avoid bruising and injury.
    3. Encourage the patient to take fluids to prevent dehydration.
    4. Assist the patient with hygiene to prevent undue fatigue.

28. An adolescent with hemophilia A wants to participate in a high school sports activity. In consultation with the health care provider, which sport would be the **best**? *(282)*
    1. Football
    2. Soccer
    3. Wrestling
    4. Golf

29. The home health nurse reads in the record that the patient has a medical diagnosis of Hodgkin's disease stage 1. Which sign/symptom would the nurse expect to see? *(288)*
    1. Abnormal single lymph node
    2. Night sweats
    3. Weight loss
    4. Alcohol-induced pain

30. Based on the nurse's knowledge of non-Hodgkin's disease, what does the nurse consider when planning care for the patient who has recently started treatment? **Select all that apply.** *(290)*
    1. Pain is likely to be localized in the spine and increases with movement.
    2. Disease is likely to be widespread and most body systems are affected.
    3. Patient could have side effects from chemotherapy.
    4. Patient and/or family may need support because prognosis is poor.
    5. Total assistance for activities of daily living is likely to be needed.

CRITICAL THINKING ACTIVITIES

Activity 1

31. A 63-year-old patient reports that her "heart is racing." She also has nausea, sore tongue, and difficulty swallowing. Upon oral examination, her tongue is smooth and erythematous. *(266)*

    a. What medical diagnosis would the nurse anticipate? _____

    b. What treatment options are available for this patient? _____

       _____

    c. After completing 2 months of treatment, the patient states she is feeling well and now plans to discontinue the treatments. How should the nurse respond to the patient?

       _____

       _____

Activity 2

32. A 32-year-old female patient has fatigue, dizziness, and pallor. Her history includes childbirth 3 months ago, a subgastrectomy 3 years ago, and hernia repair 18 months ago. Her Hgb level is 10 g/dL. *(269-271)*

    a. Based on the nurse's knowledge, what is the anticipated medical diagnosis? _____

       _____

    b. What risk factors does this patient have that support development of this disorder? _____

       _____

       _____

    c. Identify other signs and symptoms that may accompany this disorder. _____

       _____

       _____

d. Discuss six considerations for the administration of iron. _____

_____

_____

_____

_____

Activity 3

33. The nurse is caring for an older adult patient who reports bone pain that increases with movement. The medical diagnosis is multiple myeloma.

a. Discuss the benefits of ambulation and fluid for this patient. *(268)*_____

_____

b. What can the nurse do to encourage the patient to walk if he says that moving increases the pain? *(268)*

_____

_____

Activity 4

34. You are caring for a patient who is having massive hemorrhage from a wound on the thigh. The patient is in a room that is well-equipped with supplies to provide emergency care and resuscitation. There are other health care personnel on the unit. The health care provider has just ordered oxygen at 2 L/nasal cannula, 15-minute vital signs, start a peripheral IV and give a bolus of 2 L of normal saline, lower the head of the bed, apply direct pressure to the wound site then apply a pressure bandage, transfuse 1 unit of packed red blood cells, laboratory testing for platelet count and complete blood count, 1 unit of fresh frozen plasma "hold" for laboratory results, and transfer to the intensive care unit. The goals of care are 1) to stop blood loss, 2) treat for shock, and 3) restore lost volume. Discuss how you will prioritize and accomplish these orders. *(264, 265)*

a. List questions that you can ask yourself as you are formulating a plan to accomplish these orders.

_____

_____

_____

_____

b. Prioritize the health care provider's orders. _____

_____

_____

_____

_____

<table>
<tr><td>

Care of the Patient With a Cardiovascular or a Peripheral Vascular Disorder

</td><td>

chapter

8

</td></tr>
</table>

Answer Key: Textbook page references are provided as a guide for answering these questions. A complete Answer Key is provided in your Additional Learning Resources on Evolve.

TRACING A DROP OF BLOOD

1. Directions: Trace a drop of blood around the pulmonary circulatory system. Start at the superior or inferior vena cava and identify the names of the blood vessels, the chambers of the heart, and the valves of the heart. End with the drop of blood at the aorta. *(301)*

   Superior or inferior vena cava →

   _____ → _____ →

   _____ → _____ →

   _____ → _____ →

   _____ → _____ →

   _____ → _____ →

   _____ → Aorta

FIGURE LABELING

2. Directions: Label each of the coronary vessels that supply blood to the heart. *(300)*

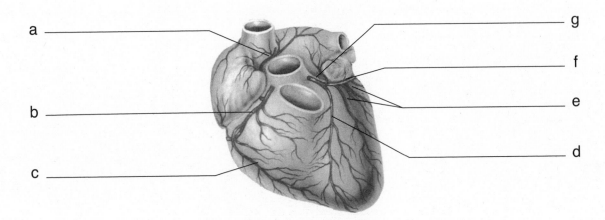

TABLE ACTIVITY

3. Directions: Complete the table with the description of what the nurse feels when palpating pulses according to the scale of: 0 to +4. *(344)*

Scale	Description of Pulse
0	
+1	
+2	
+3	
+4	

SHORT ANSWER
Directions: Using your own words, answer each question in the space provided.

4. Directions: Identify the impulse pattern of the electrical conduction system of the heart. Start at the SA node. *(299)*

   SA node →

   _____ → _____ →

   _____ → _____

5. List at least five nonpharmacologic therapies for hypertension. *(348, 349)* _____

   _____

   _____

   _____

   _____

   _____

6. What are the classic five Ps for assessing arterial occlusion? *(350)* _____

   _____

   _____

MULTIPLE CHOICE

Directions: Select the best answer(s) for each of the following questions.

7. The health care provider instructs the nurse to immediately report laboratory results to confirm the diagnosis of myocardial infarction. Which laboratory result should the nurse seek out **first**? *(304)*
   1. Creatine phosphokinase
   2. Creatine kinase
   3. Troponin T
   4. Troponin I

8. The home health nurse is reviewing the patient's laboratory results and sees that the overall serum cholesterol level is 230 mg/dL. Based on the laboratory results, which patient education topic is the nurse **most** likely to review with the patient? *(307)*
   1. Importance of ambulation and mobility
   2. Coping and stress reduction techniques
   3. Dietary sources of fat and weight reduction
   4. Methods to increase medication compliance

9. Under what circumstances would the nurse expect to observe sinus tachycardia if the patient were on a cardiac monitor? *(309)*
   1. Patient has an untreated high fever.
   2. Patient demonstrates obstructive sleep apnea.
   3. Patient faints during a bowel movement.
   4. Health care provider performs carotid massage.

10. Which physical assessment would the nurse perform to assist the health care provider in identifying atrial fibrillation? *(310)*
    1. Take a manual blood pressure on both arms.
    2. Compare bilateral peripheral pulses.
    3. Count the apical pulse for a full minute.
    4. Obtain help and check for a pulse deficit.

11. The health care provider tells that nurse the patient has occasional premature ventricular contractions (PVC). Based on this information, what would the nurse expect to observe when assessing the patient? *(311)*
    1. Shallow, rapid respiration with PVCs
    2. Chest pain when the PVCs are occurring
    3. Irregular rate and rhythm when palpating pulse
    4. Blood pressure lower than 120/80 mm Hg

12. What are the signs/symptoms of cardiac arrest? **Select all that apply.** *(314)*
    1. Pupil constriction
    2. Absence of carotid pulse
    3. Gasping respirations followed by apnea
    4. Lethargic and difficult to arouse
    5. Abrupt loss of consciousness
    6. Pallor and cyanosis

13. The health care provider is reviewing the 12-lead electrocardiogram and tells the nurse that the patient has a STEMI MI. Based on this information, what is the **priority** intervention? *(323)*
    1. Administer beta-adrenergic blocker as prescribed.
    2. Transfer to the intensive care unit.
    3. Prepare patient for thrombolytic therapy.
    4. Administer oxygen at 2 L/minute.

14. The nurse hears in report that the patient with heart failure has 4+ pitting edema in the lower extremities. Based on this information, what is the **priority** assessment that the nurse will perform? *(328)*
    1. Check for edema in the sacrum.
    2. Weigh the patient.
    3. Observe respiratory effort.
    4. Observe for jugular vein distention.

15. The patient has pulmonary edema and is prescribed furosemide. Which laboratory result is the **most** important for the nurse to monitor? *(331)*
    1. Complete blood count
    2. Electrolytes
    3. Coagulation studies
    4. Serum lipids

16. Which patient is the **most** likely candidate to meet the criteria for a cardiac transplant? *(342)*
    1. Has type 1 diabetes with end-organ damage
    2. Has heart disease stabilized by medication
    3. Has a history of mental illness
    4. Has inoperable coronary artery disease

17. The nurse is caring for a patient who is on anti-coagulant therapy. Which laboratory values are the **most** important to monitor? *(359)*
    1. Prothrombin time, International Normalized Ratio, and partial thromboplastin time
    2. Blood glucose, potassium, sodium, calcium, and magnesium
    3. Enzyme creatine kinase, creatine phosphokinase, and myoglobin
    4. B-type natriuretic peptide and troponins 1 and 2

18. Laboratory results show a low hemoglobin for a patient diagnosed with myocardial infarction. What is the **first** intervention that the nurse would perform to address this laboratory result? *(304)*
    1. Obtain an order for an intramuscular iron supplement.
    2. Help the patient to order an iron-rich meal tray.
    3. Obtain an order for type and cross for blood transfusion.
    4. Check to see that oxygen is delivered as prescribed.

19. The nurse is planning care for several patients who are scheduled to have diagnostic testing for cardiac disorders. Which patient will require postprocedural checks for peripheral pulses, color, and sensation of the extremity every 15 minutes for 1 hour? *(301)*
    1. Needs cardiac catheterization to diagnose extent of atherosclerotic heart disease
    2. Is scheduled for electrocardiogram to identify specific cardiac dysrhythmias
    3. Requires chemically induced stress electrocardiogram for poor exercise tolerance
    4. Must have positron emission tomography because of coronary artery disease

20. The nurse is discussing modifiable risk factors for cardiovascular disease with a 23-year-old patient who is currently asymptomatic. What does the nurse recommend? *(307)*
    1. Find out if any first-degree relatives had cardiovascular problems before the age of 50.
    2. Stop smoking or consider greatly reducing the number of cigarettes smoked per day.
    3. Ask the health care provider for a cholesterol-lowering drug such as simvastatin.
    4. Monitor weight and calorie intake to maintain a body mass index of 30.

21. During a discharge teaching session, the young patient voices concern about her risk for heart disease because she has diabetes mellitus. Which self-care measures would the nurse teach the patient? **Select all that apply.** *(308)*
    1. Keep the blood glucose level under control.
    2. Monitor blood pressure at home: goal less than 120/80 mm Hg.
    3. Eat a low-fat diet rich in fruits and vegetables.
    4. Exercise 3-5 times a week for at least 30 minutes.
    5. Take low-dose aspirin once a day.

22. Which psychosocial behaviors are **more** likely to be associated with increased cardiovascular symptoms? *(308)*
    1. Frequently in a hurry and generally impatient
    2. Easygoing and usually enjoys life
    3. Neat, organized, and pays attention to detail
    4. Pessimistic and generally expresses negativity

23. The patient's cardiac monitor shows a regular rhythm with a rate of 65 beats/min, P waves precede each QRS complex, QRS complexes are symmetrical and regularly spaced, and a normal T wave shows repolarization. What is the nurse's interpretation of the monitor display? *(308)*
    1. Vital signs should be immediately assessed.
    2. The monitor indicates a normal sinus rhythm.
    3. The monitor is showing a benign dysrhythmia.
    4. The patient should be assessed for chest pain.

24. The patient experiences dizziness and light-headedness while trying to pass a bowel movement. An immediate pulse check shows 45 beats/min that rapidly recovers to a regular rate of 70. What is the **most** probable cause of this episode of sinus bradycardia? *(309)*
    1. Digitalis toxicity
    2. Endocrine disturbance
    3. Intracranial tumor
    4. Vagal stimulation

25. For which dysrhythmia would a pacemaker **most** likely be necessary? *(311)*
    1. Sinus tachycardia
    2. Premature ventricular contractions
    3. Third-degree heart block
    4. Atrial fibrillation

26. The patient who had a myocardial infarction 2 weeks ago is now having frequent episodes of ventricular tachycardia. For this patient, what is the clinical significance of this dysrhythmia? *(311)*
    1. Warning sign for ventricular fibrillation
    2. Expected finding at this stage
    3. Reaction to a beta-adrenergic blocker
    4. Treatment is given only for symptoms

27. The patient is on the cardiac monitor undergoing a diagnostic procedure. Suddenly, the health care provider says, "The patient is having ventricular fibrillation." Which piece of equipment is the **most** vital? *(312)*
    1. Temporary pacemaker
    2. Defibrillator
    3. Bag-valve-mask
    4. Crash cart

28. A patient is being discharged after receiving a permanent pacemaker. What is the **best** rationale to give to the patient about refraining from sports such as tennis, swimming, golf, and weight-lifting for the first 6-8 weeks? *(315)*
    1. "First, you have to be able to climb at least two flights of stairs."
    2. "Active sports will interfere with the pacemaker's fixed mode."
    3. "These sports are too strenuous and rapidly increase the heart rate."
    4. "The arm on the pacemaker side should not be lifted over the head."

29. The patient had a percutaneous transluminal coronary angioplasty with stent placement. What type of medication is the patient **most** likely be prescribed for at least 3 months? *(319)*
    1. Digitalis preparation
    2. Diuretic
    3. Opioid pain medication
    4. Anticoagulant

30. Which instruction would the nurse give to the patient for self-administration of nitrate medications? *(321)*
    1. Refrigerate the oral tablets and nitroglycerin patches until use.
    2. Apply patches in the morning and remove them at bedtime.
    3. A burning sensation on the tongue indicates an allergic reaction.
    4. Pain relief should occur after a minimum of two doses.

31. For a patient with myocardial infarction, what symptom is the **most** important? *(322)*
    1. Diaphoresis
    2. Palpitations
    3. Pain
    4. Shortness of breath

32. A 63-year-old patient presents with fever, increased pulse, epistaxis, and joint involvement. Heart murmurs are auscultated. The patient has a history of inadequately treated childhood group A β-hemolytic streptococci pharyngitis. These findings and history are consistent with which medical diagnosis? *(336)*
    1. Cardiomyopathy
    2. Angina
    3. Left-sided heart failure
    4. Rheumatic heart disease

33. A neighbor tells the nurse that he has indigestion that has lasted 60 minutes. He tried "taking nitroglycerin, but that didn't help." What should the nurse do **first**? *(321)*
    1. Tell the neighbor to take an aspirin and then drive to the emergency department.
    2. Stay with the neighbor, assist him to remain calm, and call 911.
    3. Assess the neighbor's use of nitroglycerin and assess for other symptoms.
    4. Phone the neighbor's health care provider and ask for recommendations.

34. The health care provider is considering tissue plasminogen activator (TPA) for a patient who is having an acute myocardial infarction. The wife suddenly rushes to the nurse and says, "We forgot to tell you something." Which disclosure is a contraindication for TPA? *(323)*
    1. "My husband is a Jehovah's Witness."
    2. "My husband recently had a head injury."
    3. "He forgot to take his insulin this morning."
    4. "He had a small heart attack last year."

35. The nurse is caring for a patient who is 40 hours post–myocardial infarction. Which instruction should be given to the unlicensed assistive personnel (UAP)? *(325)*
    1. Assist the patient to ambulate in the hall three times.
    2. Check to see if the patient is too tired to get up.
    3. Encourage the patient to independently get out of bed.
    4. Help the patient get to the commode chair.

36. What is the **best** method to help a patient comply with dietary restrictions associated with atherosclerotic heart disease? *(349)*
    1. Tell him to avoid all foods that are high in fats.
    2. Remind him that total fat intake is 35%-40% of total caloric intake.
    3. Tell him to eat 10-15 grams of soluble fiber every day.
    4. Teach him how to read the nutritional labels on food products.

37. The nurse is caring for a patient who has right ventricular heart failure. After therapy, the nurse sees that the patient has lost 5 pounds of weight. Assuming that all the weight represents fluid loss, how much fluid has the patient lost? _____ L *(328)*

38. The patient with a history of heart failure tells the home health nurse, "Every night I sleep in this recliner chair. I feel better if I sleep with my head up." What will the nurse assess **first**? *(326)*
    1. Check for dependent edema in the lower extremities.
    2. Look at accessibility to the bedroom and bathroom.
    3. Assess ability to independently move and ambulate.
    4. Ask about compliance with low-sodium, low-fat diet.

39. The nurse is assessing a patient who had an embolectomy in the right lower extremity. Which assessment finding is cause for **greatest** concern? *(353)*
    1. Sudden absence of pulse in the affected extremity
    2. Capillary refill in extremity is greater than 2 seconds
    3. Affected extremity is erythematous and edematous
    4. Patient reports a tingling sensation in extremity

40. The patient arrives in the emergency department with severe dyspnea, agitation, cyanosis, audible wheezes, and a cough with blood-tinged sputum. What is the **priority** nursing action? *(334)*
    1. Obtain a blood sample for arterial blood gases.
    2. Administer oxygen.
    3. Auscultate lung sounds.
    4. Establish a peripheral IV.

41. The nurse is caring for a patient with valvular heart disease. Which task could be assigned to the UAP? *(337)*
    1. Identify activities of daily living that cause fatigue.
    2. Check meal trays for high-sodium foods.
    3. Weigh the patient at the same time every day.
    4. Explain the plan for rest periods.

42. Which disorder of the cardiovascular system places the patient at **highest** risk for the potentially life-threatening condition of cardiac tamponade? *(339)*
    1. Pericarditis
    2. Valvular heart disease
    3. Buerger's disease
    4. Endocarditis

43. Which sign/symptom indicates to the nurse that a patient with endocarditis is experiencing a serious and common complication of the disease? *(339)*
    1. Fever and chills
    2. Joint pains and aches
    3. Sudden shortness of breath
    4. Petechiae on neck and chest

44. The nurse sees an older woman sitting in the waiting room and she is crying, "My granddaughter was just diagnosed with infective endocarditis." Which therapy is the nurse **most** likely to explain to the grandmother? *(341)*
    1. Prosthetic valve replacement
    2. Intensive antibiotic therapy
    3. Complete bedrest
    4. Anticoagulation therapy

45. Which patient should be counseled about the risk of cardiomyopathy related to lifestyle choices? *(341)*
    1. High-risk sexual behavior
    2. Poor intake of dietary fiber
    3. Use of "crack" cocaine
    4. Social consumption of alcohol

46. The patient had a recent cardiac transplant. Which intervention is required for posttransplant care? *(342)*
    1. Immunosuppressive therapy
    2. Pericardiocentesis
    3. Percutaneous transluminal angioplasty
    4. Contact isolation

47. A younger patient has had several blood pressure readings that are consistently staying around 130/80 mm Hg. What treatments and/or advice should be given to this patient? *(346)*
    1. Diuretics and low-sodium diet
    2. Beta-adrenergic blockers and weight loss
    3. Angiotensin II receptor blockers and low-fat diet
    4. Lifestyle change and routine health appointments

48. The nurse is caring for a patient who has peripheral arterial disease with burning pain in the right leg that occurs at rest. Which intervention will the nurse use? *(352)*
    1. Elevate the leg on a pillow.
    2. Use a covered ice compress.
    3. Place the leg in a dependent position.
    4. Encourage aerobic exercise for circulation.

49. A patient receives a prescription for anticoagulant medication for treatment of arterial emboli. What dietary information should the nurse give? *(353)*
    1. Do not increase intake of dark-green vegetables because of vitamin K.
    2. Take extra dairy products to ensure calcium intake and vitamin D.
    3. Eat fruits such as citrus and bananas that provide potassium.
    4. Avoid eating saturated fats by limiting use of butter, oils, and red meats.

50. The nurse is monitoring a patient who is waiting for diagnostic testing to determine if he has an aortic aneurysm. The patient suddenly reports severe chest pain. He becomes pale, weak, and confused. His pulse is 130 beats/min and blood pressure is 85/50 mm Hg. What should the nurse do **first**? *(355)*
    1. Call the health care provider.
    2. Put the patient in a supine position.
    3. Assess pain and give opioid medication.
    4. Establish a patent peripheral IV.

51. The nurse is caring for a postsurgical patient. Which intervention is the **most** important in preventing venous thrombosis in the legs? *(360)*
    1. Applying elastic compression stockings
    2. Elevating the lower extremities
    3. Ensuring early ambulation and mobility
    4. Measuring the calf circumference daily

CRITICAL THINKING ACTIVITIES

Activity 1

52. A 56-year-old man with a history of angina arrives in the emergency department seeking care. He reports crushing chest pain that radiates down his left shoulder and arm. "The pain is more severe and has lasted longer than a typical angina episode." *(321-325)*

a. What data should the nurse collect? _____

_____

_____

_____

b. What does the nurse anticipate this patient's medical diagnosis will be? _____

_____

c. What are the goals of the medical management of this patient? _____

_____

d. Identify at least six nursing interventions for this patient's care._____

_____

_____

_____

_____

_____

_____

Activity 2

53. A 43-year-old Native American woman presents with "heaviness in her chest." She reports that it radiates down her left inner arm. Her medical history includes childbirth, pancreatitis, and hypertension. The medical diagnosis of angina is made. *(316, 317)*

a. What risk factors for heart disease does the patient have? _____

_____

_____

b. What medications are used to treat angina? _____

_____

_____

Activity 3

54. A home health nurse is caring for a 73-year-old man who has heart failure. He has been hospitalized twice for exacerbations, but is currently stable and able to live independently in his own home.

   a. What changes related to aging would the nurse expect to find for this patient's cardiac system? *(306)*

   _____

   _____

   b. What are common signs and symptoms of heart failure? *(329)* _____

   _____

   _____

   c. Identify medication classes that are used in the medical management of heart failure. *(330-331)*

   _____

   _____

   d. Discuss patient teaching points for heart failure. *(334)* _____

   _____

   _____

Activity 4

55. The nurse is working in an ambulatory walk-in clinic in an urban area. Many of the patients are homeless and the clinic staff sees many patients who have venous stasis ulcers.

   a. What is the pathophysiology of stasis ulcers and why are the homeless at risk for this disorder? *(361)*

   _____

   b. Describe how the nurse would use PATCHES to assess venous disorders. *(344)* _____

   _____

   _____

   _____

   c. Identify the signs and symptoms of venous stasis ulcers. *(361)* _____

   _____

   _____

   d. Review the treatment options available for venous stasis ulcers and suggest how the nurse can assist homeless patients to obtain care. *(361)*

   _____

   _____

   _____

Activity 5

56. Check the cupboards of an older relative or patient (or your own cupboards) and read nutritional labels on packages. Determine if a typical day's use of the products on the shelf would meet the nutritional restrictions for someone on a cardioprotective diet. (Don't forget to check condiments, if they are likely to be included in daily use.) Record your findings and the recommendations that you would make about the choice of food products. *(327)*

_____

_____

_____

_____

_____

_____

_____

_____

Care of the Patient With a Respiratory Disorder

Answer Key: Textbook page references are provided as a guide for answering these questions. A complete Answer Key is provided in your Additional Learning Resources on Evolve.

MATCHING

Medication Used for Respiratory Disorders

Directions: Match the medication used for a respiratory disorder on the left to the associated characteristic (action, side effect, or nursing implication) on the right. Indicate your answers in the spaces provided. (395-397)

	Medication		Actions, Side Effects, or Nursing Implications
_____	1. Acetylcysteine	a.	Vasoconstrictor used for nasal congestion
_____	2. Salmeterol	b.	Beta$_1$- and beta$_2$-receptor agonist; could cause tachycardia, palpitations, angina, chest pain, myocardial infarction, dysrhythmias, hypertension, restlessness, agitation, anxiety
_____	3. Prednisone		
_____	4. Epinephrine		
_____	5. Albuterol	c.	Bronchodilator; can cause anxiety, restlessness, insomnia, headache, seizures, tachycardia, dysrhythmias
_____	6. Isoniazid	d.	Mucolytic agent; also used as antidote in acetaminophen overdose
_____	7. Oxymetazoline		
_____	8. Theophylline	e.	Used in prevention of exercise-induced asthma
_____	9. Rifampin	f.	Antiinflammatory agent; do not discontinue medication abruptly; dosage must be tapered slowly
_____	10. Zafirlukast		
		g.	"Rescue therapy;" short-acting inhaled beta$_2$-agonist
		h.	Antitubercular agent; monitor liver function tests
		i.	For long-term treatment of asthma
		j.	Antitubercular agent; long-term therapy

TABLE ACTIVITY

11. Directions: Complete the table by filling in the normal values for an arterial blood gas. *(377)*

pH:	
Pa$_{CO_2}$:	
Pa$_{O_2}$:	
HCO$_3^-$:	
Sa$_{O_2}$:	

MULTIPLE CHOICE

Directions: Select the best answer(s) for each of the following questions.

12. The inner linings of the pharynx and the eustachian tube are continuous. In children, this normal anatomical structure contributes to what common disorder? *(380)*
    1. Asthma
    2. Epistaxis
    3. Laryngitis
    4. Ear infections

13. If the epiglottis fails to perform its intended function, how would this affect the patient? *(369)*
    1. Increased risk for aspiration
    2. Increased incidence of throat infections
    3. Decreased respiratory drive
    4. Decreased forced expiratory volume

14. The nurse is assessing a newborn who was brought to the clinic for the initial well-baby physical. The newborn demonstrates a respiratory rate of 50 breaths/min. How does the nurse interpret this data? *(372)*
    1. Newborn's respiratory rate suggests a hypermetabolic state, such as fever.
    2. Newborn must be immediately taken to resuscitation area for respiratory distress.
    3. Newborn's respiratory rate is within the expected range for developmental age.
    4. Newborn's respiratory rate is borderline high and should be closely monitored.

15. The patient has increased intracranial pressure and the nurse knows that the medulla oblongata and pons of the brain have a role in respiration. If increased intracranial pressure is uncontrolled and excessive, what is the potential adverse effect on respiratory function? *(372)*
    1. Respiratory infection
    2. Respiratory arrest
    3. Respiratory edema
    4. Respiratory acidosis

16. The nurse is assessing a child who is "having an asthma attack." Which assessment finding is cause for **greatest** concern? *(373)*
    1. Audible wheezing on expiration
    2. Subjective sensation of chest tightness
    3. Increased pulse and respiratory rate
    4. Substernal and clavicular retractions

17. A neighbor tells the nurse that he is "pretty healthy and doesn't take any medications" but seems to have nosebleeds that are occurring more frequently. What does the nurse suggest **first**? *(379)*
    1. "To stop bleeding, hold pressure on the lower nose for 10-15 minutes."
    2. "Let's check your blood pressure for the next several mornings."
    3. "Make an appointment to have your clotting times checked."
    4. "Have your health care provider examine your nasal septum."

18. What is an **early** sign of cancer of the larynx? *(383)*
    1. Pain radiating to the ear
    2. Difficulty swallowing
    3. Feeling of a lump in the throat
    4. Progressive or persistent hoarseness

19. Which persons should be advised to get pneumococcal vaccination? **Select all that apply.** *(399)*
    1. 18-month-old child with no known health problems
    2. 25-year-old nurse with no known health problems
    3. 80-year-old with chronic conditions who lives in a nursing home
    4. 35-year-old with diabetes mellitus that is well-controlled with insulin
    5. 40-year-old in good general health, who travels outside the United States
    6. 19-year-old who smokes two packs of cigarettes per day

20. The nurse is caring for a patient who sustained rib fractures during a car accident. The patient reports sudden sharp chest pain over the fracture area, with difficulty breathing. Which assessment finding supports the nurse's suspicion of pneumothorax? *(407)*
    1. Bilateral wheeze during inspiration and expiration
    2. Decreased breath sounds over the affected area
    3. Coarse crackles heard in early inspiration
    4. Dry creaking and grating when breath is held

21. The patient had a permanent tracheostomy several months ago. At this point, what is the **priority** concern? *(385)*
    1. Breathing independently and safely.
    2. Secreting adequate amounts of mucus.
    3. Being unable to produce normal speech.
    4. Swallowing without choking or gagging.

22. A patient with a chronic lung disorder comes to the clinic and tells the nurse, "I feel like I am getting sick again." What questions would the nurse ask? **Select all that apply.** *(372)*
    1. "How's your breathing? Can you describe it?"
    2. "Are you coughing? Can you describe the cough?"
    3. "When did you first notice the worsening of symptoms?"
    4. "What were your last arterial blood gas results?"
    5. "Do you use oxygen at home? If so, does it help?"
    6. "Have you noticed a change in your ability to do routine activities?"

23. The patient arrives at the emergency department and displays significant respiratory distress. Which objective finding is generally regarded as a **late** sign of respiratory distress? *(373)*
    1. Shows increased respiratory rate
    2. Has adventitious breath sounds
    3. Assumes orthopneic position
    4. Demonstrates flaring of nostrils

24. A patient was brought to the emergency department because he was involved in a motor vehicle accident. The patient shows mild respiratory distress and expansion of the right side of the chest is decreased compared to the left. The history and data are indicative of which disorder? *(407)*
    1. Pleural effusion
    2. Pneumothorax
    3. Empyema
    4. Pulmonary edema

25. Which patient has the **greatest** need for a helical computed tomography scan? *(374)*
    1. A disoriented older patient who may have a pulmonary embolus
    2. A toddler who might have swallowed a metallic foreign body
    3. A patient who requires a sample of lymph node tissue for biopsy
    4. A patient who was exposed to tuberculosis several decades ago

26. The nurse is caring for a patient who had a bronchoscopy. Which task can be delegated to the unlicensed assistive personnel (UAP)? *(375)*
    1. Give clear fluids after checking for the gag reflex.
    2. Assist the patient to a semi-Fowler's position.
    3. Report signs of laryngeal edema such as stridor.
    4. Check sputum for signs of hemorrhage.

27. The patient needs a thoracentesis for therapeutic removal of fluid. Which position should the nurse help the patient to assume for the procedure? *(376)*
    1. Seated on the bed; head and arms resting on a pillow placed on an overbed table
    2. Placed in a supine position with the anterior lateral chest draped for ready access
    3. Positioned in a recumbent prone position with head resting on forearms and hands
    4. Situated in a side-lying position on affected side and uncovered to the waist

28. The nurse hears in handover report that 1600 mL of fluid was removed during the therapeutic thoracentesis procedure. What is the **most** important intervention that the nurse will plan to do? *(403)*
    1. Perform routine postprocedure assessments.
    2. Increase the fluid intake to compensate for the loss.
    3. Watch for signs and symptoms of pulmonary edema.
    4. Follow up to get the results of the fluid specimen.

29. When an arterial blood gas is obtained from a patient who is taking warfarin, what special consideration is needed? *(377)*
    1. The dietary therapy associated with the drug is likely to alter the results.
    2. The drug increases fragility of the vessels, so the specimen is hard to obtain.
    3. The drug alters the amount of oxygen that hemoglobin can carry.
    4. The clotting time is prolonged; pressure is held for 20 minutes on the puncture site.

30. The nursing student uses an automatic blood pressure cuff to take vital signs. To be efficient, the student simultaneously attaches the pulse oximeter to the patient's same hand. The pulse oximeter reading is below 90%. What should the student do **first**? *(378)*
    1. Report the findings to the nurse or instructor.
    2. Redo the pulse oximeter reading on the other hand.
    3. Assess the patient for shortness of breath.
    4. Document the finding in the patient's record.

31. A patient was treated for epistaxis with nasal packing saturated with 1:1000 epinephrine. During the postprocedure assessment, the nurse notices that the patient swallows frequently. Which question should the nurse ask? *(379)*
    1. "Does your throat feel swollen or painful?"
    2. "Would you like some cool fluids to drink?"
    3. "Is blood running down the back of your throat?"
    4. "Are you tasting epinephrine in your throat?"

32. What is likely to be included in the discharge instructions for a patient who was treated for epistaxis? **Select all that apply.** *(379)*
    1. Use a vaporizer.
    2. Use saline nose drops.
    3. Apply nasal lubricants.
    4. Take aspirin for pain as needed.
    5. Vigorously blow to remove clots.
    6. Avoid inserting foreign objects into nose.

33. What is the nurse's role in allergy testing? *(381)*
    1. Uses a lancet to prick the skin with different allergens
    2. Evaluates the response to different allergens
    3. Advises the patient about allergens to avoid
    4. Determines schedule for retesting questionable allergens

34. The nurse is eating in a restaurant. At a nearby table, several men are talking, laughing, drinking alcohol, and eating steak. Suddenly, the nurse hears, "Hey! Are you all right?" Which behavior signals a need to intervene for choking? *(383)*
    1. Vigorous coughing
    2. Running from the room
    3. Hand over throat
    4. Waving hands frantically

35. A patient is diagnosed with viral laryngitis. Which discharge instruction is the **most** important to relieve the inflammation and edema of the vocal cords? *(388)*
    1. Use a mild analgesic such as acetaminophen for pain.
    2. Complete the full course of antibiotics.
    3. Rest the voice; communicate with gestures or by writing.
    4. Suck on throat lozenges to promote comfort.

36. The nurse is performing a rapid strep screen. What is the rationale for obtaining two throat swabs? *(388)*
    1. The first swab is likely to be contaminated, so a backup swab is needed.
    2. If the rapid strep test is negative, the second swab is sent for culture.
    3. The second swab is given to the patient, in case the rapid strep is positive.
    4. The first and second swabs are grown in different types of culture media.

37. A patient comes to the clinic and reports decreased appetite, generalized malaise, and a decreased sense of smell. Gentle palpation over the sinus area elicits pain. Which piece of equipment should the nurse obtain so the health care provider can do some diagnostic testing during the physical examination? *(389)*
    1. Tongue blade
    2. Percussion hammer
    3. Penlight
    4. Cotton-tipped applicator

38. A patient is diagnosed with acute bronchitis. Although the patient is instructed to increase fluids to 3000-4000 mL per day, which fluid is specifically not recommended because of the respiratory condition? *(390)*
    1. Coffee
    2. Soda
    3. Orange juice
    4. Milk

39. What is the **primary** problem for the health care team in identifying potentially life-threatening respiratory disorders such as Legionnaires' disease, severe acute respiratory syndrome, and anthrax? *(391, 392)*
    1. They are agents used in global germ warfare.
    2. The percentage of morbidity and mortality is high.
    3. They require isolation because transmission is airborne.
    4. At first, symptoms are similar to other respiratory disorders.

40. What is the **major** problem for patients who are being treated for tuberculosis? *(398)*
    1. All the patient's contacts must be identified and treated.
    2. Infection control measures are complex and expensive.
    3. Many have rapid disease progression with mortality rates up to 89%.
    4. Drug therapy lasts 6-9 months and about 50% of patients are noncompliant.

41. A patient recently diagnosed with peripherally located lung cancer reports he is experiencing severe chest pain. Based on the nurse's knowledge of the pathophysiology of this pain, which therapy does the nurse anticipate? *(372, 408)*
    1. Bronchodilators
    2. Thoracentesis
    3. Mechanical ventilation
    4. Corticosteroids

42. The patient is diagnosed with pleurisy. During auscultation of the lungs, what is the nurse **most** likely to hear? *(373)*
    1. Interrupted crackling or bubbling sounds more common on inspiration
    2. Deep, loud, low, coarse sound (like a snore) during inspiration or expiration
    3. Dry, creaking, grating, with a machinelike quality loudest over anterior chest
    4. High-pitched, musical, whistlelike sound during inspiration or expiration

43. A patient being treated for atelectasis has been prescribed acetylcysteine. What is the purpose of this medication? *(395)*
    1. Reduce the risk of infection
    2. Dilate the bronchioles
    3. Enhance the cough reflex
    4. Reduce viscosity of secretions

44. For a patient with a chest tube, which task could be delegated to the UAP? *(404)*
    1. Assist to ambulate with water-seal below the level of the chest.
    2. Check to make sure that all connections are secure and intact.
    3. Observe for and report hypoventilation or increased dyspnea.
    4. Assess quantity and quality of drainage in the collection chamber.

45. The nurse is reviewing the admission orders for a patient who was stabilized in the emergency department and then admitted for a diagnosis of pulmonary edema. Which order is the nurse **most** likely to question? *(410)*
    1. Oxygen 2 L per nasal cannula
    2. Notify provider with all blood gas results
    3. IV normal saline at 250 mL per hour
    4. Place on telemetry monitor

46. A patient is admitted for venous thrombosis in the left leg. He is in good spirits during the AM assessment, but later in day he reports feeling mildly short of breath with a sense of impending doom. What should the nurse do **first**? *(412)*
    1. Obtain an order for an arterial blood gas.
    2. Check the vital signs and pulse oximeter reading.
    3. Assess the left leg for warmth, redness, or swelling.
    4. Alert the RN about possible pulmonary embolus.

47. Which patient has the **highest** mortality risk related to acute respiratory distress syndrome? *(413)*
    1. Was diagnosed and treated for sepsis 5 days ago
    2. Had direct trauma to chest during a fight 10 days ago
    3. Has a history of chronic obstructive pulmonary disease
    4. Has been treated for asthma since early childhood

48. Which instruction would the nurse give to the UAP about assisting the patient who has emphysema to accomplish activities of daily living (ADLs)? *(418)*
    1. Divide hygienic care into short sessions with 90 minutes of rest between.
    2. Defer the hygienic care until the patient has better activity tolerance.
    3. Assess the patient's response to ambulating and shorten walks accordingly.
    4. Perform range-of-motion exercises, unless the patient declines them.

49. For a patient with chronic bronchitis, what is the physiologic cause of polycythemia? *(419)*
    1. Medication side effect
    2. Dehydration and fluid shifting
    3. Nutritional deficiency
    4. Compensation for chronic hypoxemia

50. For a patient with newly diagnosed asthma, what is the **best** rationale for assessing the home environment? *(420)*
    1. Identify any activity intolerance related to the design of the home.
    2. Assess the safety of the environment related to the use of home oxygen.
    3. Identify stimulants or allergens that are triggering the asthma attacks.
    4. Evaluate the need for a home health aide to accomplish ADLs.

51. The home health nurse reads in the patient's record that he has smoked for the past 30 years and was recently diagnosed with emphysema. Which assessment finding does the nurse expect as the **primary** manifestation? *(416)*
    1. Dyspnea on exertion
    2. Copious thick sputum
    3. Barrel-chest appearance
    4. Bulbous, shiny fingernails

CRITICAL THINKING ACTIVITIES

Activity 1

52. A 34-year-old man comes to the clinic for fatigue and headaches in the morning. The nurse's assessment reveals he is 5'9" and weighs 293 pounds. His blood pressure is 155/92 mm Hg. His health history reveals elevated blood pressure, hernia repair, appendectomy, and recent injuries suffered from a motor vehicle accident after falling asleep while driving. During the interview, his wife states he should never be tired because he snores so loudly at night that she is the one who is kept awake. *(381, 382)*

    a. Based on the nurse's knowledge, what medical diagnosis is anticipated? _____

    _____

    b. What risk factors and elements of the patient's personal history support this diagnosis? _____

    _____

    _____

    _____

    c. Discuss the medical management of this condition. _____

    _____

    _____

    _____

    _____

Activity 2

53. A 72-year-old man is transferred from the nursing home to the hospital with a diagnosis of viral pneumonia. *(400, 401)*

   a. What signs and symptoms are associated with this type of pneumonia? _____

   _____

   _____

   b. What diagnostic tests can the nurse expect to be completed for this patient? _____

   _____

   _____

   c. What types of medications may be prescribed for this patient?_____

   _____

   _____

   d. Identify nursing assessments that should be performed for this patient._____

   _____

   _____

Activity 3

54. a. Discuss factors that may influence medication compliance for tuberculosis patients. *(394, 398)*

   _____

   _____

   _____

   _____

   b. Suggest interventions to increase compliance. *(398)* _____

   _____

   _____

   _____

   _____

   _____

   _____

   _____

Activity 4

55. The nurse hears in report that the patient has a closed chest drainage system. *(396)*

    a. What nursing assessments should be performed for this patient? _____

       _____

       _____

    b. How should the tubing and the chest drainage system be positioned? _____

       _____

       _____

    c. How does the nurse interpret the absence of tidaling (air bubbling) in the water seal chamber?

       _____

       _____

    d. What does constant bubbling in the water seal chamber indicate? _____

       _____

       _____

Care of the Patient With a Urinary Disorder

Answer Key: Textbook page references are provided as a guide for answering these questions. A complete Answer Key is provided in your Additional Learning Resources on Evolve.

SHORT ANSWER

Directions: Using your own words, answer each question in the space provided.

1. What are the three major functions of the nephron? *(429)*

   a. _____

   b. _____

   c. _____

2. Summarize the three phases of urine formation. *(430)*

   a. _____

   b. _____

   c. _____

3. Identify at least three life span considerations for older adults related to the urinary system. *(432)*

   _____

   _____

   _____

4. What are the major functions of the kidneys? *(431)* _____

   _____

   _____

   _____

   _____

   _____

   _____

TABLE ACTIVITY

Directions: Complete the table below by supplying the normal range for urinalysis results and identify at least one factor that could influence the results. The first constituent is completed for you. (433)

5. Urinalysis

Constituent	Normal Range	Influencing Factors
Color	Pale yellow to amber	Diabetes insipidus, biliary obstruction, medications, diet
Turbidity		
Odor		
pH		
Specific gravity		
Glucose		
Protein		
Bilirubin		
Hemoglobin		
Ketones		
Red blood cells		
White blood cells		
Casts		
Bacteria		

FIGURE LABELING

6. Directions: Identify the ileal conduit, stoma, and anastomosis on the figure below. *(473)*

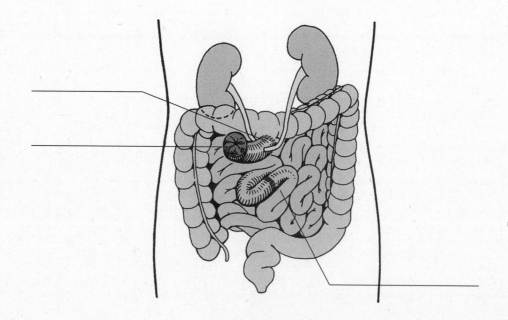

MULTIPLE CHOICE

Directions: Select the best answer(s) for each of the following questions.

7. The nurse is reviewing laboratory results for a young healthy patient who has no known health problems. The blood urea nitrogen (BUN) level is 26 mg/dL. What question is the nurse **most** likely to ask to clarify this laboratory result? *(434)*
   1. "Have you had an exposure to a sexually transmitted infection?"
   2. "Did you eat or drink anything before you had the blood drawn?"
   3. "Do you have a family history of diabetes or liver problems?"
   4. "Are you having any problems with starting the urine stream?"

8. The nurse hears in report that the patient is in the diuretic phase of acute renal failure. What assessment findings does the nurse expect? *(465)*
   1. BUN is over 50 mg/dL, serum creatinine is greater than 5 mg/dL, urine output is less than 30 mL/hour.
   2. BUN and serum creatinine levels begin to normalize and urinary output is 1 to 2 L/24 hours.
   3. Glomerular filtration rate rises and kidneys are at normal or near-normal function.
   4. BUN and serum creatinine levels rise and urinary output is less than 400 mL/24 hours.

9. The nurse is caring for several patients who need diagnostic testing for problems associated with the urinary system. Which patient is **most** likely to need insertion of an indwelling urinary catheter prior to having the procedure? *(435)*
   1. Patient needs an intravenous pyelogram for possible hydronephrosis.
   2. Patient needs renal venography for possible dysfunction of venous drainage.
   3. Patient needs a renal ultrasonography for possible congenital anomaly.
   4. Patient needs a voiding cystourethrogram for possible abnormal urethra.

10. The nurse is caring for a patient who returned to the unit after a cystoscopy for diagnosis of a disorder of the urinary bladder. Which post-procedure assessment would be considered a normal finding? *(435)*
    1. Increased output and low specific gravity
    2. Urinary retention and bladder distention
    3. Blood-tinged urine at the first void
    4. Mild flank pain and low-grade fever

11. Which staff member should not be assigned to care for a patient who has returned from a renal scan that used a radionuclide tracer substance? *(436)*
    1. Unlicensed assistive personnel (UAP) who is in the first trimester of pregnancy
    2. LPN/LVN who is taking medication for a urinary tract infection
    3. RN who is immunosuppressed secondary to a splenectomy
    4. UAP who has allergies to iodine, seafood, and latex

12. Which patient is **most** likely to benefit from patient education pamphlets about urodynamic studies and rectal electromyography? *(436)*
    1. Patient has renal cancer, staging yet to be determined.
    2. Patient has risk for polycystic kidney disease.
    3. Patient has urinary incontinence related to neurologic disorder.
    4. Patient has signs/symptoms of chronic glomerulonephritis.

13. The nurse is caring a patient who is prescribed furosemide for acute renal failure. What nursing interventions are related to the medication and acute renal failure? **Select all that apply.** *(437)*
    1. Keep accurate intake and output (I&O) records.
    2. Assess BUN and serum electrolytes.
    3. Teach the patient to avoid overuse of salt.
    4. Monitor for flank and abdominal pain.
    5. Record and monitor daily morning weights.

14. Which breakfast tray is the **best** example of foods that adhere to the acid-ash diet? *(439)*
    1. Blueberry pancakes with maple syrup and tea
    2. Coffee, orange juice, and granola with raisins
    3. Whole-grain toast, boiled egg, and prunes
    4. Low-fat milk, banana, and peanut butter toast

15. What instructions would the nurse give to the UAP about the care of a patient who has an indwelling catheter and urinary collection bag? **Select all that apply.** *(440)*
    1. Never rest the collecting bag on the floor.
    2. Cleanse the perineum from front to back with mild soap and warm water, then pat dry.
    3. Inspect the catheter entry site for blood, exudate, or other signs of infection.
    4. Avoid kinks or compression of the drainage tubing.
    5. Assist the patient to ambulate; hold drainage bag below the catheter insertion site.

16. A patient is prescribed sulfamethoxazole-trimethoprim. What is the **most** important point to stress in teaching the patient about this medication? *(446)*
    1. Expect an increase in urination and try to take the medication in the morning.
    2. Complete the full course of medication even if feeling better after a day or two.
    3. The medication makes the urine a bright orange color, but this is harmless.
    4. Drink at least 2000 mL of water every day to prevent crystal precipitation.

17. For patients with diabetes mellitus or starvation states, urinalysis will show the abnormal presences of ketones. What is the underlying pathophysiology for this abnormality? *(431)*
    1. Fatty acids are rapidly catabolized.
    2. Glucose is converted to ketones.
    3. Insulin levels are excessive.
    4. Glucose is transformed into fat.

18. Which patient condition is **most** likely to result in casts in the urine specimen? *(463)*
    1. Type 1 diabetes mellitus
    2. Stress incontinence
    3. Acute pyelonephritis
    4. Ureter structure trauma

19. The nurse sees that the urine specific gravity results are 1.000 g/mL. Which patient condition is **most** likely to result in this abnormal finding? *(433)*
    1. Diabetic ketoacidosis
    2. Hyperemesis gravidarum
    3. Diabetes insipidus
    4. Febrile with poor skin turgor

20. Identify the renal disorders associated with an abnormal elevation in serum creatinine. **Select all that apply.** *(434)*
    1. Stress incontinence
    2. Glomerulonephritis
    3. Pyelonephritis
    4. Acute tubular necrosis
    5. Acute renal failure

21. A 49-year-old man's prostate-specific antigen (PSA) result is 9.5 ng/mL. Which condition(s) could be associated with this result? **Select all that apply.** *(434)*
    1. Had a recent prostate biopsy
    2. Could be related to prostate cancer
    3. Suggests urinary tract infection
    4. Indicative of prostatitis
    5. Within normal limits for age

22. The nurse is planning care for several patients who will have diagnostic testing for urinary disorders. Which procedure is going to require the **most** time for postprocedural care? *(435)*
    1. Kidney-ureter-bladder radiography
    2. Intravenous pyelogram
    3. Renal angiography
    4. Renal ultrasonography

23. During a urodynamic study, a patient is given bethanechol, a cholinergic drug. What is the expected effect of the medication? *(436)*
    1. Relaxes the patient
    2. Reduces urine production
    3. Stimulates the atonic bladder
    4. Increases the uptake of dye

24. What instructions would the nurse give to the UAP for assisting a patient for the first 24 hours after a renal biopsy? *(436)*
    1. Assist the patient to ambulate to the bathroom.
    2. Ask the patient about dizziness before ambulating.
    3. Withhold all foods and fluids for 24 hours.
    4. Remind the patient about bedrest for 24 hours.

25. The nurse is reviewing medication prescriptions for a patient with advanced end-stage renal disease. The nurse would question the use of which type of medication? *(438)*
    1. Antiemetic
    2. Antipruritic
    3. Vitamin supplement
    4. Osmotic diuretic

26. The nurse is caring for several older male patients who have problems with urinary disorders. Which patient is the **best** candidate for an external condom? *(440)*
    1. Has Alzheimer's disease and recently pulled out an indwelling catheter
    2. Has urge incontinence and functional incontinence related to a hip fracture
    3. Has a urinary tract infection and is currently taking antibiotics
    4. Has an enlarged prostate and occasionally has trouble starting the stream

27. What is an **early** sign of bladder cancer? *(456)*
    1. Change in voiding pattern
    2. Dusky yellow-tan or gray skin color
    3. Painless, intermittent hematuria
    4. Difficult starting the stream of urine

28. The nurse sees that the patient who is being discharged is prescribed spironolactone. Which laboratory result will the nurse verify before the patient goes home? *(437)*
    1. Urinalysis
    2. Potassium level
    3. White cell count
    4. Blood urea nitrogen

29. A patient with benign prostatic hyperplasia (BPH) tells the nurse that he uses over-the-counter (OTC) medications. Which medication is likely to create additional problems related to the BPH? *(442)*
    1. Acetaminophen
    2. Diphenhydramine
    3. Vitamin K supplement
    4. Iron supplement

30. Which patient is **most** likely to benefit from learning about Kegel exercises? *(443)*
    1. Experiences loss of urine during sneezing and lifting
    2. Has urinary retention secondary to chronic infection
    3. Has urge incontinence due to advanced Parkinson's disease
    4. Has a spastic bladder due to upper motor neuron lesion

31. The nurse and UAP are aware that no tension should be placed on urinary catheters; however, the nurse should reinforce this principle for which patient? *(462)*
    1. Has a suprapubic catheter for long-term management
    2. Has a three-way catheter for continuous bladder irrigation
    3. Has an indwelling catheter after reconstruction of urethra
    4. Has a catheter and urometer for hourly measurements

32. For patients with nephrotic syndrome, which signs/symptoms is the nurse **most** likely to observe? *(462)*
    1. Periorbital edema, pitting edema in legs, and crackles in lungs
    2. Sore throat or skin infection with fever and malaise
    3. Burning with urination, low back pain, hematuria, and fatigue
    4. Dysuria, weak stream, and increasing pain with bladder distention

33. The patient with acute glomerulonephritis is placed on bedrest. Which vital sign is of **primary** interest as an indicator of the success of the therapy? *(464)*
    1. Temperature
    2. Pulse rate
    3. Respiratory rate
    4. Blood pressure

34. What is an indicator of chronic glomerulonephritis? *(464)*
    1. Residual urine
    2. Albumin in the urine
    3. Ketones in the urine
    4. Prostate-specific antigen

35. A student nurse is assessing the function of an arteriovenous fistula after a dialysis treatment. When would the supervising nurse intervene? *(469)*
    1. Flushes with saline using strict aseptic technique.
    2. Palpates a thrill and auscultates for a bruit.
    3. Assesses the distal pulses and checks for sensation.
    4. Asks the patient about pain or discomfort at the site.

CRITICAL THINKING ACTIVITIES

Activity 1

36. A 42-year-old patient has a history of frequent urinary tract infections and is admitted to the unit with a diagnosis of pyelonephritis. *(449, 450)*

    a. What signs and symptoms would the nurse anticipate the patient to demonstrate? _____

    _____

    _____

    b. Discuss the diagnostic tests that may be used in the treatment of the patient and the probable results.

    _____

    _____

Activity 2

37. A patient comes to the emergency department for severe flank pain, nausea, and vomiting. The patient reports that the pain starts in the flank area and radiates to the groin and inner thigh. A urinalysis reveals the presence of hematuria. *(452, 453)*

    a. What medical diagnosis does the nurse anticipate?_____

    _____

    b. Discuss the conservative and invasive techniques that may be used in the management of this condition.

    _____

    _____

    c. After successful treatment, the nurse is preparing the patient for discharge. Discuss long-term preventive management options. Include diet and medications.

    _____

    _____

Activity 3

38. A 53-year-old man was in a motor vehicle accident 4 days ago. He sustained serious trauma with hypovolemia that was treated in the emergency department. He has been diagnosed with acute renal failure and is currently in the oliguric phase. *(465, 466)*

   a. What potential clinical manifestations should the nurse be aware of when completing the nursing assessment?

   _____

   _____

   b. Discuss the three phases of acute renal failure. _____

   _____

   _____

   _____

   c. The patient's wife asks if she can bring him a hamburger and fries from a local fast-food restaurant. How will the nurse respond?

   _____

   _____

Activity 4

39. A 22-year-old woman seeks care at the health care provider's office complaining of burning with urination, perineal pain, and blood-tinged urine. She is diagnosed with a urinary tract infection. *(438, 447)*

   a. Why are women more prone to urinary tract infections compared to men? _____

   _____

   b. What other signs and symptoms may be present? _____

   _____

   c. What medical treatments can be anticipated in the management of this patient? _____

   _____

   d. What self-care measures should the nurse suggest to the patient to prevent urinary tract infections?

   _____

   _____

   _____

Care of the Patient With an Endocrine Disorder

Answer Key: Textbook page references are provided as a guide for answering these questions. A complete Answer Key is provided in your Additional Learning Resources on Evolve.

MATCHING

Directions: Match the hormone produced by the gland to the action on the target organ. Indicate your answer in the space provided.

Hormone (Endocrine Gland)

_____ 1. oxytocin (posterior pituitary) *(479)*

_____ 2. antidiuretic (posterior pituitary) *(479)*

_____ 3. thyroxine (thyroid) *(481)*

_____ 4. calcitonin (thyroid) *(481)*

_____ 5. parathormone (parathyroid) *(481)*

_____ 6. mineralocorticoids (adrenal cortex) *(481)*

_____ 7. glucocorticoids (adrenal cortex) *(481)*

_____ 8. epinephrine (adrenal medulla) *(482)*

_____ 9. norepinephrine (adrenal medulla) *(482)*

_____ 10. insulin (pancreas) *(482)*

_____ 11. glucagon (pancreas) *(482)*

_____ 12. melatonin (pineal) *(482)*

Action on Target Organ

a. Causes the kidneys to conserve water by decreasing the amount of urine produced

b. Promotes the release of milk and stimulates uterine contractions during labor

c. Decreases blood calcium levels by causing calcium to be stored in the bones

d. Growth and development; metabolism

e. Involved in glucose metabolism; provides extra reserve energy in times of stress; exhibits antiinflammatory properties

f. Causes the heart rate and blood pressure to increase

g. Increases the concentration of calcium in the blood and regulates phosphorus in the blood

h. Water and electrolyte balance; indirectly manages blood pressure

i. Secreted in response to decreased levels of glucose in the blood

j. Inhibits reproductive activities by inhibiting the gonadotropic hormones

k. Combines with epinephrine to produce "fight-or-flight" response

l. Secreted in response to increased levels of glucose in the blood

FIGURE LABELING

13. Directions: Label the figure below by indicating the position of the glands of the body. *(479)*

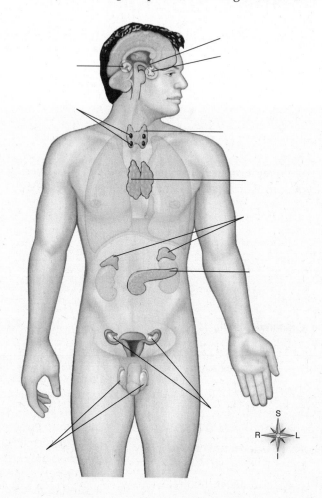

TABLE ACTIVITY

14. Directions: Complete the table below with the correct information about different types of insulin. *(510)*

Type of Insulin	Injection Time (Before Meal)	Risk Time for Hypoglycemic Reaction	Onset of Action	Duration
Lispro (Humalog)				
Regular Humulin R Novolin R ReliOn R				
NPH/Regular Mix 70/30 Humulin Mix 70/30				
Glargine (Lantus)				

MULTIPLE CHOICE

Directions: Select the best answer(s) for each of the following questions.

15. Which electrolyte disorder is **most** likely to trigger early symptoms of syndrome of inappropriate antidiuretic hormone (SIADH)? *(488)*
    1. Hypokalemia
    2. Hyponatremia
    3. Hypercalcemia
    4. Hyperglycemia

16. What instructions are given to the unlicensed assistive personnel (UAP) about the care of a patient with hypothyroidism? **Select all that apply.** *(493)*
    1. Report frequency of bowel movements; straining; or small, hard stools.
    2. Allow extra time for physical care so the patient doesn't feel rushed.
    3. Make sure the patient does not become chilled during bathing.
    4. Observe patient's activity cycle and perform interventions accordingly.
    5. Encourage patient to select fruits, vegetables, and whole grains from menu.

17. A 53-year-old patient has just been informed that he has type 2 diabetes. Which patient education pamphlet is the nurse **most** likely to prepare for this patient? *(508)*
    1. "A Step-by-Step Approach to Self-Administration of Insulin"
    2. "Side Effects of Common Oral Hypoglycemic Medications"
    3. "How to Manage Your Diabetes during Stress or Illness"
    4. "Using Exercise and Diet Modification for Weight Loss"

18. Which endocrine disorder is associated with the long-term complications of retinopathy; nephropathy; amputation of lower extremity; and cardiovascular conditions such as heart disease, hypertension, and stroke? *(504)*
    1. Hyperparathyroidism
    2. Diabetes insipidus
    3. Cushing's syndrome
    4. Diabetes mellitus

19. Which patient always needs to have an emergency kit with 100 mg of IM hydrocortisone, syringes, and instructions for use? *(502)*
    1. Patient has pheochromocytoma and is not a good candidate for the necessary surgery.
    2. Patient has Addison's disease and is having stress related to death of a family member.
    3. Patient has type 1 diabetes and is prone to episodes of sudden-onset hypoglycemia.
    4. Patient has hyperthyroidism and is having trouble tolerating the antithyroid drugs.

20. In the care of a patient with diabetic ketoacidosis, the nurse is **most** likely to contact the health care provider for clarification of which prescription? *(509)*
    1. IV normal saline at 1000 L/hr until urinary output is at least 30 mL/hr
    2. Perform fingerstick for blood glucose level every hour
    3. Insert urinary catheter with urometer; monitor I&O every hour
    4. 100 units NPH insulin in 500 mL normal saline; titrate to blood glucose

21. What are **early** signs/symptoms of hypothyroidism? **Select all that apply.** *(493)*
    1. Weight gain
    2. Difficulty concentrating
    3. Constipation
    4. Infertility
    5. Depression
    6. Mood swings

22. The nurse is talking to a 31-year-old woman who was recently diagnosed with acromegaly. The woman says, "My career is over. I'll become so hideous, I'm sure that I'll get fired." What is the **most** therapeutic response? *(483)*
    1. "You have talents and abilities; surely those qualities will be considered."
    2. "Why don't you wait and cross that bridge when you come to it?"
    3. "You are thinking about how your life and career might change."
    4. "Let's talk about what you could do to enhance your appearance."

23. The school nurse is taking height and weight measurements for all children at the beginning of the school year. Measurement for one of the students shows a deviation over two percentile levels from the median. What should the nurse do? *(485)*
    1. Call the parents and ask about the child's birth weight and growth patterns.
    2. Contact the parents and suggest they take the child to the health care provider.
    3. Recheck the child's height and weight once a month for the next several months.
    4. Track the child's growth over time and compare findings to siblings and classmates.

24. Which nursing interventions should be employed for a patient with diabetes insipidus? **Select all that apply.** *(487)*
    1. Assessment of skin turgor
    2. Daily weight measurement
    3. Fluid restriction
    4. Monitor I&O
    5. Frequent ambulation

25. Which patient has the **greatest** risk for developing SIADH? *(488)*
    1. Has malignant cancer
    2. Has dormant tuberculosis
    3. Suffered head trauma
    4. Received opioid medication

26. The nurse is caring for a patient who is diagnosed with SIADH. Which assessment finding indicates that the disorder has progressed to neurologic involvement? *(488)*
    1. An increased urge to drink fluids
    2. A decrease in serum sodium
    3. Progression to shock symptoms
    4. A change in mental status

27. For the patient with SIADH, the health care provider orders fluid restriction. Which finding **best** indicates that the therapy is working? *(488)*
    1. Patient reports that he feels better.
    2. Vital signs are at patient's baseline.
    3. Serum sodium is gradually increased.
    4. Diuretics are gradually discontinued.

28. The nurse is caring for a patient who had a thyroidectomy. Which routine postoperative intervention would the nurse clarify with the health care provider? *(491)*
    1. Inspect dressing for bleeding and drainage.
    2. Give clear liquids; progress to soft diet.
    3. Encourage coughing and deep-breathing.
    4. Observe surgical site for signs of infection.

29. The health care provider tells the nurse that the patient needs diagnostic testing for possible hyperthyroidism. What symptoms is the patient **most** likely to exhibit? *(489)*
    1. Weight loss, increased appetite, and nervousness
    2. Intolerance to cold, constipation, and lethargy
    3. Skeletal pain, pain on weight-bearing, and paranoia
    4. Polyphagia, polydipsia, and polyuria

30. The nurse is reviewing the patient's medication prescriptions and sees that the patient takes levothyroxine. Which laboratory result will indicate efficacy of therapy? *(484)*
    1. Blood glucose less than 250 mg/dL
    2. Normalization of urine specific gravity
    3. Gradual improvement of serum sodium level
    4. Normalization of thyroid-stimulating hormone level

31. The nurse is caring for a patient who had a thyroidectomy 6 hours ago. The patient exhibits thyroid crisis and receives treatment. Which outcome statement indicates that the goals of therapy were met? *(492)*
    1. Patient's sodium level is normalized, and fluid intake equals urinary output.
    2. Patient's low blood glucose returns to 60 mg/dL and mental status is at baseline.
    3. Patient displays euthyroid, blood pressure and temperature are at baseline.
    4. Patient's cortisol level returns to baseline, hypotension is resolved.

32. The health care provider tells the nurse that the patient has a firm, fixed, small, rounded, painless nodule that was palpated on the thyroid gland. The nurse prepares to support the patient when the provider informs about the need for diagnostic testing for which disorder? *(495)*
    1. Myxedema
    2. Colloid goiter
    3. Thyroid cancer
    4. Cretinism

33. The nurse is caring for a patient who has a pathologic fracture secondary to hyperparathyroidism. Which food needs to be taken off the patient's breakfast tray? *(497)*
    1. Glass of whole milk
    2. White toast with jam
    3. Sugared cereal flakes
    4. Fried egg with bacon

34. Why is furosemide (diuretic) prescribed for a patient with hyperparathyroidism? *(497)*
    1. Preserve existing kidney function
    2. Decrease fluid retention and edema
    3. Encourage the elimination of serum calcium
    4. Decrease blood pressure

35. The LPN is assisting an RN with a patient who needs emergency administration of calcium gluconate for hypoparathyroid tetany. The RN is preparing the medication. What task should the LPN/LVN perform under the supervision of the RN? *(497)*
    1. Assess the patient for medication allergies.
    2. Place the patient on electrocardiographic monitoring.
    3. Assess the patency of the intravenous access.
    4. Verify the prescription for calcium gluconate.

36. For patients who have hypoparathyroidism, why is it important for the nurse to encourage foods such as soy milk, white rice, jam, honey, lemon-lime soda, cucumbers, lettuce, peppers, tomatoes, and non-organ meats? *(498)*
    1. These foods supply extra calcium, which is needed to treat hypocalcemia.
    2. These foods are low in phosphorus, and serum phosphorus is elevated.
    3. These foods supply vitamin D, which improves the absorption of calcium.
    4. These foods are low in fat and will not be metabolized into ketones.

37. Urine excreted by a patient with diabetes insipidus will exhibit which characteristics? *(486)*
    1. Dilute, with a specific gravity of 1.005–1.030
    2. Dilute, with a specific gravity of 1.001–1.005
    3. Concentrated, with a specific gravity of 1.005–1.030
    4. Concentrated, with a specific gravity of 1.001–1.005

38. What is the pathophysiology of simple goiter? *(494)*
    1. The growth is harmless, like a fluid-filled cyst that can be drained.
    2. There is fluid retention in the face and neck because of a blockage.
    3. The gland usually enlarges because of lack of iodine in the diet.
    4. The surrounding tissue becomes inflamed and swollen because of infection.

39. Cortisol is responsible for what bodily function? *(481)*
    1. Regulates sodium levels
    2. Regulates potassium levels
    3. Provides energy during stress
    4. Responds to decreased glucose levels

40. What type of insulin administration is indicated in the management of hyperglycemia related to diabetic ketoacidosis? *(509)*
    1. Glargine insulin given subcutaneously
    2. Humulin N insulin given subcutaneously
    3. NPH 70/30 given intravenously
    4. Regular insulin given intravenously

41. A patient is diagnosed with corticosteroid-induced Cushing's syndrome. Which statement by the patient indicates a need for additional teaching? *(500)*
    1. "I would like to try a dose reduction."
    2. "I am going to stop taking the medication."
    3. "I prefer trying a gradual discontinuation."
    4. "I am changing to the alternate-day regimen."

42. The patient with Cushing's syndrome has high risk for skin breakdown. What instructions will the nurse give to the UAP to prevent skin impairment? *(500)*
    1. Handle very gently to prevent bruising and ecchymosis.
    2. Assess for signs of erythema, edema, or infection.
    3. Frequently wash the skin to prevent irritation.
    4. Assist females to remove extra hair with a safety razor.

43. The nurse is caring for a patient who is admitted with Addison's disease. During the AM assessment, the nurse notes very high temperature and orthostatic hypotension. Laboratory results show hyponatremia and hyperkalemia. How does the nurse interpret these findings? *(501)*
    1. These are expected findings for this disorder; continue routine assessment.
    2. The frequency of assessment should be increased; reassess status every 1-2 hours.
    3. These are signs of impending addisonian crisis; notify the health care provider.
    4. These should be documented as abnormal findings; compare data for trends.

44. The principal manifestation of pheochromocytoma is severe hypertension. What other symptoms are likely to accompany the excessive secretion of catecholamines (i.e., epinephrine and norepinephrine)? *(502)*
    1. Lethargy, constipation, and depression
    2. Tachycardia, diaphoresis, and anxiety
    3. Kussmaul's respiration, hypotension, and drowsiness
    4. Excessive thirst, increased urine output, and lethargy

45. Which diagnostic test is the **best** for monitoring long-term compliance for patients with diabetes mellitus? *(506)*
    1. Fasting blood glucose (FBG)
    2. Postprandial (after a meal) blood glucose (PPBG)
    3. Patient self-monitoring of blood glucose (SMBG)
    4. Glycosylated hemoglobin (HbA$_{1c}$)

46. Which patient needs to test the urine for ketones as part of self-care management? *(507)*
    1. Gestational diabetic who has started insulin
    2. Type 2 diabetic who is preparing to exercise
    3. Type 1 diabetic who has a febrile infection
    4. An older diabetic who cannot perform SMBG

47. The pharmacy delivers a bag of insulin to be delivered as a piggyback infusion. The label says that 100 units of regular insulin is mixed in 500 mL of normal saline. How many mL would be required to deliver 3 units per hour? _____ mL/hr *(518)*

48. A nurse hears in shift report that a diabetic patient has had nothing by mouth (NPO) since midnight for a surgical procedure that should happen this morning. On assessment, the patient is irritable and his skin is cool and clammy. His blood glucose is 45 mg/dL. What should the nurse do **first**? *(517)*
    1. Give the patient some juice and a peanut butter sandwich.
    2. Administer 50% glucose per emergency protocol.
    3. Call the operating room and cancel the procedure.
    4. Call the health care provider and inform about findings.

CRITICAL THINKING ACTIVITIES

Activity 1

49. A 19-year-old woman seeks care because of excessive thirst, hunger, and fatigue. She reports she has not been able to sleep all night for the past few weeks because of needing to go to the bathroom.

   a. Based on the nurse's knowledge, what medical diagnosis is anticipated? *(505)* _____

   _____

   b. What other clinical manifestations may occur in this patient? *(505, 506)* _____

   _____

   _____

   _____

   _____

   c. Describe what the nurse will teach the patient about administering insulin. *(513)* _____

   _____

   _____

   _____

   _____

   d. Upon realizing this condition is not curable, the patient asks what acute and long-term complications are associated with diabetes. How will the nurse respond to this inquiry? *(504, 515)*

   _____

   _____

   _____

   _____

Activity 2

50. The parents of a 6-year-old boy report to the health care provider with concerns about their son's height. They report that he is the smallest child in the school. The parents are of normal stature. Assessment reveals that the child is indeed significantly small for his age. *(485, 486)*

   a. What diagnostic tests can be anticipated? _____

   _____

   _____

   b. What other clinical manifestations may be exhibited by a child with dwarfism? _____

   _____

   _____

c. Another question voiced by the parents is the future implications for their child. How will the nurse respond?

_____

_____

_____

d. What medical treatment will be prescribed for this patient? _____

_____

_____

Activity 3

51. Discuss considerations for older adults related to endocrine disorders. *(515)* _____

_____

_____

_____

_____

Activity 4

52. Why should patients with endocrine disorders be advised to wear medical alert jewelry? *(487, 511)*

_____

_____

_____

_____

Care of the Patient With a Reproductive Disorder

Answer Key: Textbook page references are provided as a guide for answering these questions. A complete Answer Key is provided in your Additional Learning Resources on Evolve.

FIGURE LABELING

1.   Directions: Label the parts of the female reproductive system. *(529)*

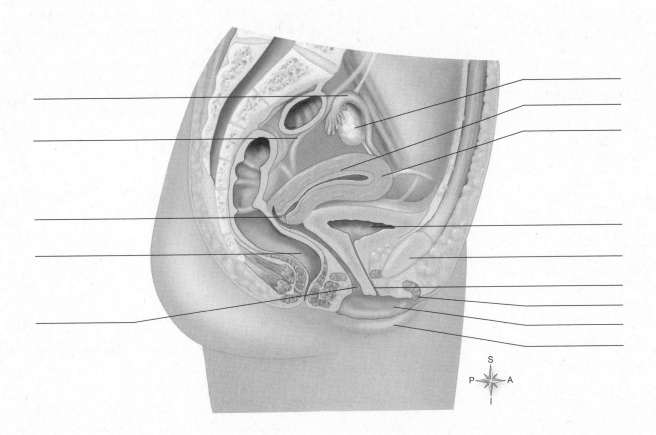

MATCHING

Directions: Match the birth control method with the description. Indicate your answers in the spaces provided. (588)

	Method		**Description**
_____	2.	combination pill	a. Take two within 72 hours of coitus; repeat if vomiting occurs; take second dose 12 hours later
_____	3.	morning-after pill	
_____	4.	progestin-only pill	b. Consists of a thin flexible rod, which is inserted subdermally
_____	5.	medroxyprogesterone	
_____	6.	Implanon	c. Rubber thimble-shaped shield covering cervix, held in place by suction
_____	7.	diaphragm	d. Device inserted into uterus; flexible object made of plastic or copper wire
_____	8.	cervical cap	e. No pill-free days
_____	9.	male condom	f. Double-ring system fitted into vagina up to 8 hours before intercourse
_____	10.	female condom	
_____	11.	intrauterine device	g. Contains both estrogen and progesterone
_____	12.	rhythm method	h. Only drug given by injection every 3 months
_____	13.	tubal sterilization	i. Dome-shaped latex cap with flexible metal ring
_____	14.	hysterectomy	j. Thin rubber sheath fitting over erect penis
_____	15.	vasectomy	k. Bilateral surgical ligation and resection of ductus deferens
			l. Crushing, ligating, clipping, or plugging of fallopian tubes
			m. Requires periodic abstinence during fertile portion of menstrual cycle
			n. Surgical removal of uterus; 100% effective

SHORT ANSWER

Directions: Using your own words, answer each question in the space provided.

16. Identify three functions of the organs of the male reproductive system. *(527)*

a. _____

b. _____

c. _____

17. What are three questions that the nurse would use to take a brief sexual history assessment? *(533)*

a. _____

b. _____

c. _____

18. What are the most common disturbances related to menstruation? *(539)*

a. _____

b. _____

c. _____

d. _____

e. _____

19. What are four main factors that contribute to sexually transmitted infections being among the world's most common communicable diseases? *(581)*

a. _____

b. _____

c. _____

d. _____

FIGURE LABELING

20. Directions: Label the lymph nodes of the axilla. *(567)*

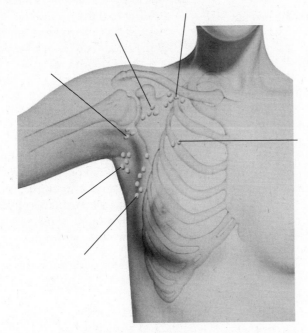

TABLE ACTIVITY

21. Directions: Using the 5 Ps, complete the table below with questions that the nurse would ask to assess risk factors for sexually transmitted infections. *(582)*

Assessment of Risk Factors for Sexually Transmitted Infections Using the 5 Ps

5 Ps	Questions to Ask
Past STIs	
Partners	
Practices	
Prevention	
Pregnancy	

MULTIPLE CHOICE

Directions: Select the best answer(s) for each of the following questions.

22. The school nurse is reviewing the health records of children. Which parents should be contacted to follow up with the health care provider about their daughter's reproductive health? *(539)*
    1. Girl was 9 years old when menarche started.
    2. Girl was 15 years old when menarche started.
    3. Girl is 11 years old and there is no breast development.
    4. Girl is 16 years old and menarche has not started.

23. Which person is the **best** example of fulfilling a gender role? *(532)*
    1. Young woman pursues an intimate same-sex relationship.
    2. A 3-year old boy plays with a toy truck that's just like daddy's.
    3. Middle-aged man enjoys wearing his wife's clothes.
    4. Young woman investigates sex change procedures.

24. Which woman should be advised to have an annual clinical breast examination and mammogram? *(567)*
    1. 18-year-old woman who has two children
    2. 65-year-old woman who is obese
    3. 40-year-old woman with average risk
    4. 35-year-old woman with average risk

25. Which illnesses can result in actual inability to function sexually? **Select all that apply.** *(534)*
    1. Diabetes mellitus
    2. End-stage renal disease
    3. Primary syphilis
    4. Hypertension
    5. Spinal cord injuries

26. Which woman needs to be advised to have an annual Pap smear? *(535)*
    1. A 17-year-old who has been sexually active since age 14
    2. A 19-year-old who has never been sexually active
    3. A 31-year-old who had three normal consecutive Pap smears
    4. A 25-year-old who had a hysterectomy for traumatic injury

27. A 23-year-old woman reports not having a period for several months. The health care provider tells the nurse that the patient needs diagnostic procedures/tests. Which procedures/tests does the nurse anticipate will be **first**? *(540)*
    1. Serum hormone studies such as estradiol or prolactin
    2. Ultrasound and computed tomography scan
    3. Genetic testing and family history review for cancers
    4. Pregnancy test and pelvic examination

28. In caring for men who have had diagnostic testing of the reproductive system, the nurse would provide the comfort measures of scrotal support and an ice application for which diagnostic test? *(538)*
    1. Semen analysis
    2. Prostatic smear
    3. Testicular biopsy
    4. Prostate-specific antigen

29. Following a cystoscopy, which finding would be considered normal? *(538)*
    1. Elevated temperature
    2. Decreased urinary output
    3. Pink-tinged urine
    4. Low back pain

30. For which condition is the nurse **most** likely to use a heat application as a comfort measure? *(541)*
    1. Amenorrhea
    2. Dysmenorrhea
    3. Menorrhagia
    4. Metrorrhagia

31. The nurse is interviewing a patient who reports that her menstrual periods seem heavier than usual. Which question(s) would the nurse ask? **Select all that apply.** *(543)*
    1. "How many days have you had menstrual flow?"
    2. "How many days would your period typically last?"
    3. "How many pads or tampons are you saturating per day?"
    4. "How frequently would you normally change a pad/tampon?"
    5. "Do you take aspirin or other anticoagulant medications?"
    6. "Have you recently started a rigorous exercise program?"

32. The nurse is planning patient education for several patients. Which patient is **most** likely to need instructions on how to keep a journal for two or three menstrual cycles, which includes symptoms and activities that relate to the menses? *(544, 545)*
    1. 24-year-old woman reports irritability, fatigue, and depression with headache, backache, and breast tenderness
    2. 57-year-old woman reports feelings of being unwanted, fear of aging, hot flashes, and dyspareunia
    3. 18-year-old woman reports colicky pain prior to menses that radiates to perineum and back
    4. 34-year-old woman reports feeling angry, frustrated, and saddened because of inability to conceive

33. Which disorder is **most** likely to be treated with an antidepressant medication? *(544)*
    1. Premenstrual syndrome
    2. Premenstrual dysphoric disorder
    3. Pelvic inflammatory disease
    4. Polycystic ovary syndrome

34. A 56-year-old woman reports that she went through menopause 3 years ago but has started to menstruate again and she wonders if she should start using birth control. What should the nurse say? *(544)*
    1. "Resuming birth control is a good idea if you don't want to get pregnant."
    2. "Pregnancy is probably not likely since you went through menopause 3 years ago."
    3. "Vaginal bleeding after menopause is not expected. See your gynecologist."
    4. "Does your current flow look like it did before you went through menopause?"

35. What is the physiologic rationale that supports use of calcium and vitamin D supplements for postmenopausal women? *(546)*
    1. These supplements are an alternative to hormone replacement therapy to relieve hot flashes.
    2. Decreased bone density occurs with menopause; calcium and vitamin D support bone health.
    3. Calcium and vitamin D mimic estrogen and progesterone in their structure and function in the body.
    4. Postmenopausal women are more likely to decrease active exercises that contribute to bone health.

36. For most menopausal women, which symptom/condition could be relieved by using a water-soluble lubricant? *(547)*
    1. Pruritus
    2. Dysmenorrhea
    3. Dyspareunia
    4. Procidentia

37. The woman is undergoing a tubal insufflation test. Which outcome suggests that the fallopian tubes are blocked? *(538)*
    1. No pain or other symptoms are experienced during the test.
    2. The patient experiences shoulder pain during the test.
    3. A high-pitched bubbling is auscultated over the abdomen.
    4. A radiographic film shows free gas under the diaphragm.

38. A 57-year-old male patient confides in the nurse that he doesn't feel as productive or sexually powerful as he used to. What should the nurse say **first**? *(537)*
    1. "I understand how you feel; aging makes us feel like time is slipping away."
    2. "You'll be okay. Look at all the things you have accomplished so far."
    3. "What factors are contributing to the changes that you see in yourself?"
    4. "Let's talk about ways that you can cope with your loss of sexual power."

39. The nurse is reviewing the medication lists for several patients. Which combination of medications must be immediately brought to the attention of the provider? *(548)*
    1. Sildenafil citrate and nitroglycerin tablets
    2. Vitamin B_6 supplement and ibuprofen
    3. Cefoxitin and steroids
    4. Danazol and vitamin E supplement

40. The nurse places the patient with pelvic inflammatory disease in Fowler's position. What is the rationale for using this position for this patient? *(552)*
    1. Facilitate respiratory effort
    2. Prevent aspiration
    3. Facilitate vaginal drainage
    4. Decrease strain on the abdomen

41. What is an **early** manifestation of toxic shock syndrome? *(553)*
    1. Decreased urine output
    2. Flulike symptoms
    3. Desquamation of palms
    4. Hypotension

42. What advice does the nurse give about tampon use to prevent toxic shock syndrome? *(554)*
    1. Use an applicator to insert super-absorbent tampons.
    2. Wash hands thoroughly after inserting a tampon.
    3. Tampons should be changed every 8 hours.
    4. Alternate the use of tampons with use of pads.

43. The nurse hears in report that the patient has a vesicovaginal fistula. What assessment finding does the nurse expect? *(555)*
    1. Trickling of urine from the vagina
    2. Expulsion of feces and flatus from the vagina
    3. Patient report of "something coming down"
    4. Vaginal flow similar to regular menses

44. Radiation has been scheduled for a patient diagnosed with breast cancer. When developing the plan of care, when should the nurse anticipate radiation will take place? *(570)*
    1. Radiation will begin within 72 hours after surgery.
    2. Radiation will begin within 1 week after surgery.
    3. Radiation will begin 2-3 weeks after surgery.
    4. Radiation will begin 4-6 weeks after surgery.

45. What is an advantage of brachytherapy over traditional radiation therapy for early stage breast cancer ? *(570)*
    1. Is more cost-effective
    2. Will take less time to complete
    3. Is associated with fewer side effects
    4. Uses a lower dosage of radiation

46. Anemia is a side effect associated with chemotherapy. Which medication may be prescribed to manage this complication? *(570)*
    1. Epoetin alfa
    2. Prochlorperazine
    3. Granisetron
    4. Ondansetron

47. Tamoxifen has been prescribed for a patient diagnosed with breast cancer. Which characteristics are associated with tamoxifen? **Select all that apply.** *(571)*
    1. Inhibits the growth-stimulating effects of estrogen
    2. Hormonal agent of choice for postmenopausal women
    3. Used to manage recurrent breast cancer
    4. Used to prevent breast cancer in high-risk individuals
    5. Used for women desiring continued fertility

48. An autologous bone marrow transplant is planned for a patient with breast cancer. Which action will the nurse perform? *(571)*
    1. Maintain radiation safety while caring for the patient before the transplant.
    2. Prepare the patient to donate bone marrow, from which stem cells will be harvested.
    3. Administer chemotherapy after the stem cell transplant is completed.
    4. Reinforce explanation of plasmapheresis that is performed on the donor stem cells.

49. A 22-year-old woman who has a history of cervical dysplasia is scheduled for a conization procedure to remove a small eroded area on her cervix. What nursing care is appropriate for this procedure? *(535)*
    1. Assess for allergies to seafood or iodine.
    2. Monitor for bleeding after the procedure.
    3. Encourage fluids prior to the procedure.
    4. Remind to refrain from using deodorants.

50. Which medications are used in the treatment of dysmenorrhea? **Select all that apply.** *(541)*
    1. Oral contraceptives
    2. Ibuprofen
    3. Fluconazole
    4. Calcium
    5. Naproxen sodium

51. Endometrial cancer usually affects postmenopausal women. What is generally the **first** sign? *(561)*
    1. Vague abdominal discomfort
    2. Offensive vaginal exudate
    3. Flulike symptoms
    4. Abnormal uterine bleeding

52. Which piece of equipment is the nurse **most** likely to obtain to assist the health care provider in differentiating hydrocele from a cancerous testicular mass? *(578)*
    1. Doppler
    2. Flashlight
    3. Hemoccult card
    4. Culture swab

53. What is the treatment of choice for primary syphilis? *(583)*
    1. Penicillin
    2. Acyclovir
    3. Valacyclovir
    4. Tetracycline

54. The health care provider tells the nurse that the male patient has gonorrhea. What signs/symptoms would the nurse expect to observe? *(584)*
    1. Painful, erythematous, vesicular eruptions on or in the genitalia or rectum
    2. Painless erosion or papule with superficial ulceration and a scooped-out appearance
    3. Scanty white or clear exudate, burning around meatus, urinary frequency, and mild dysuria
    4. Urethritis, dysuria, frequent urination, pruritus, and purulent penile discharge

55. A patient and partner each received a prescription for a 7-day course of oral metronidazole for the treatment of trichomoniasis. In addition to sexual abstinence during treatment and completion of all prescribed antibiotics, what instructions will the nurse give about the medication? *(542)*
    1. Notify provider of weight gain of 5 lb or more per week.
    2. Avoid drinking alcohol during therapy.
    3. Take medication with a full glass of water.
    4. Watch for and report edema in the extremities.

56. The nurse is chaperoning a group of adolescent girls on a camping trip. One of the girls goes to lie down in the tent, "because I'm on my period." On assessment, the girl has flulike symptoms, an elevated temperature, sore throat, diarrhea, headache, and a diffuse rash. Which question is the nurse **most** likely to ask? *(553)*
    1. "Is there any chance you could be pregnant? If, so have you passed any clots or tissue?"
    2. "Are you sexually active? If so, have you been using barrier protection against disease?"
    3. "Are you wearing a tampon? If so, when was the last time you changed it?"
    4. "Is this a typical period for you? If so, how do you usually manage these symptoms?"

57. A patient who has a pessary reports foul-smelling discharge, vaginal irritation, and painful sexual intercourse. Which question should the nurse ask? *(557)*
    1. "Have you been using vaginal douching?"
    2. "Are you having burning with urination?"
    3. "When was the pessary last cleaned?"
    4. "Do you use spermicidal for birth control?"

CRITICAL THINKING ACTIVITIES

Activity 1

58. A 20-year-old patient reports to the family planning clinic for painful, erythematous vesicles on her genitals. She is scared and voices many questions and concerns about her condition. *(581, 582)*

    a. Based on the nurse's knowledge, what is the anticipated medical diagnosis? _____

    _____

    _____

    _____

    _____

    _____

    b. What treatment options and interventions are available to the patient? _____

    _____

    _____

    _____

    c. What should be included in the patient education?_____

    _____

    _____

    _____

    _____

Activity 2

59. The nurse is preparing to discuss menstruation with a group of preteen girls. The nurse will include the following teaching points. *(539)*

    a. At what age do girls typically begin menstruation? _____

    b. How long does a typical menstrual period last and approximately how much blood is lost during the average menstrual period?

    _____

    _____

    c. What will the nurse tell the girls about personal hygiene?_____

    _____

    _____

    _____

Activity 3

60. The nurse is originally from a very small farming town in the western United States, but after graduating, she decides to work in an urban clinic that serves an inner-city community in a very large city in the eastern part of the United States.

a. What are the risk factors for the clinic population that are likely to contribute to reproductive disorders? *(580)*

_____

_____

_____

_____

b. What can the nurse do to prepare herself to help patients that may have gender identity beliefs or sexual practices that are different from her own? *(532, 533)*

_____

_____

_____

_____

Activity 4

61. Discuss the emotional impact for a couple who is undergoing diagnostic testing for infertility. *(549, 550)*

_____

_____

_____

_____

_____

_____

_____

_____

Care of the Patient With a Visual or Auditory Disorder

Answer Key: Textbook page references are provided as a guide for answering these questions. A complete Answer Key is provided in your Additional Learning Resources on Evolve.

FIGURE LABELING

1. Directions: Label the anatomy of the eye. *(597)*

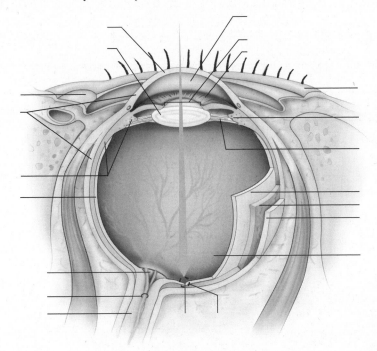

SHORT ANSWER

Directions: Using your own words, answer each question in the space provided.

2. What four basic processes are necessary to form an image? *(598)*

   a. _____

   b. _____

   c. _____

   d. _____

3.   Define the following types of blindness. *(600)*

   a.   Total blindness: _____

   b.   Functional blindness: _____

   c.   Legal blindness: _____

4.   Briefly define the six types of hearing loss. *(626)*

   a. _____

   b. _____

   c. _____

   d. _____

   e. _____

   f. _____

5.   Identify the four taste sensations and the locations of the taste bud receptors. *(638)*

   a. _____

   b. _____

   c. _____

   d. _____

FIGURE LABELING

6.   Directions: Label the anatomy of the external, middle, and inner ear. *(623)*

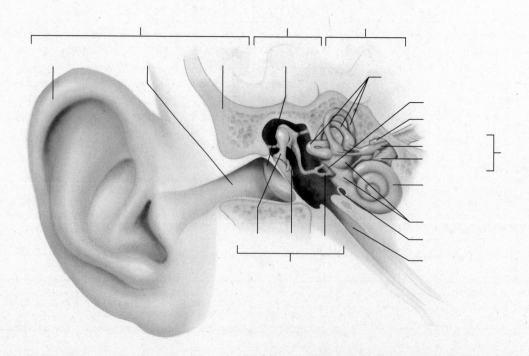

MULTIPLE CHOICE

Directions: select the best answer(s) for each of the following questions.

7. The patient is given a functional vision assessment (American Foundation for the Blind), and even with corrective lenses, the patient is unable to complete the distance task. For which task is the patient **most** likely to need assistance? *(601)*
   1. Going up and down stairs
   2. Reading a label on a medication container
   3. Driving to a clinic appointment
   4. Preparing and cooking dinner

8. The patient shows loss and deterioration in the automated perimetry test. Which activity is the patient **most** likely to have difficulty with? *(599)*
   1. Reading a newspaper or book
   2. Participating in a basketball game
   3. Looking at a laptop computer screen
   4. Going on a moonlight stroll down the street

9. Which diagnostic test requires an assessment of allergies to seafood or iodine? *(599)*
   1. Snellen test
   2. Slit-lamp examination
   3. Fluorescein angiography
   4. Tonometry

10. The nurse is reviewing the medication prescriptions for several patients with disorders of the eye. The nurse would question the health care provider about the use of corticosteroids for which patient? *(607)*
    1. Patient had cataract surgery
    2. Patient has dry eye with inflammation
    3. Patient had a corneal transplant
    4. Patient needs treatment for keratitis

11. The nurse hears in the shift report that the patient has diplopia. Which task will be the **most** difficult for the patient? *(598)*
    1. Sitting upright in bed
    2. Reading an information brochure
    3. Listening to a radio broadcast
    4. Eating a sandwich with fries

12. The nurse is orienting the patient to the hospital environment. He is just learning to use a cane as an assistive device for partial blindness. Which interventions would the nurse use? **Select all that apply.** *(601)*
    1. Walk silently beside the patient, so that he can hear environmental noises.
    2. Suggest that the cane be used to identify borders or objects in pathways.
    3. Walk behind the patient, so that the pathway is clear for him/her.
    4. Advise to walk slowly, especially since the environment is unfamiliar.
    5. Describe the general layout of the room and the adjacent hallway.

13. For which eye condition are patients **most** likely to try self-treatment with over-the-counter eyewear? *(603)*
    1. Astigmatism
    2. Strabismus
    3. Myopia
    4. Hyperopia

14. A patient with myopia is thinking about having refractory surgery to correct the problem. What should the patient do prior to the surgery? *(603)*
    1. Arrange to take at least 2 weeks off from work for recuperation.
    2. Stop wearing contact lenses for 1-2 weeks before surgical evaluation.
    3. Stop taking any medications for at least 2 days before the surgery.
    4. Use sterile hydrating eyedrops for at least 2 weeks prior to surgery.

15. The nurse's teenage son tells him that his contact lens fell out while he was hanging out in the park with his friends, so he used saliva to clean it off. Which question should the nurse ask? *(604)*
    1. "Did you ask if anybody had contact lens solution or a lens case?"
    2. "You know you are not supposed to do that, don't you?"
    3. "So what are you planning to do if that happens again?"
    4. "Do you think glasses would be a better option for you?"

16. The nurse has a 10-year-old daughter who wants to invite two friends for a sleepover. Part of the entertainment for the night is to do "glamour makeovers." What should the nurse do? *(620)*
    1. Tell the daughter that sharing eye makeup contributes to eye infections.
    2. Call the other parents and see if the friends currently have eye infections.
    3. Purchase three makeup kits from the drugstore and supervise the activity.
    4. Teach the children how to use a fresh cotton-tip applicator for application.

17. The home health nurse is supervising a parent who is demonstrating care for her child's conjunctivitis. The nurse would intervene if the mother performed which action? *(606)*
    1. Used a clean washcloth to wipe away the secretions
    2. Applied a warm compress with a clean cloth for comfort
    3. Instilled the eyedrops in the lower conjunctival sac
    4. Taped an eyepad loosely over the affected eye

18. For a patient who is diagnosed with keratitis, which common symptom differentiates this disease from other inflammatory eye diseases? *(606)*
    1. Elevated body temperature
    2. Severe eye pain
    3. Presence of halos or flashes
    4. Low white cell count

19. A patient has recently been diagnosed with keratoconjunctivitis sicca and a dry mouth. Which immune disorder is likely to be associated with this diagnosis and symptom? *(607)*
    1. Sjögren's syndrome
    2. Acquired immunodeficiency syndrome
    3. Rheumatoid arthritis
    4. Type 1 diabetes mellitus

20. With Sjögren's syndrome, what would the nurse expect the patient to report? *(607)*
    1. Seeing floaters in the field of vision
    2. Color blindness
    3. Feeling worse in the morning
    4. Sensation of grit in the eyes

21. What are the signs/symptoms of ectropion? **Select all that apply.** *(608)*
    1. Tearing
    2. Redness of sclera
    3. Thick eye discharge
    4. Corneal dryness
    5. Outward turning of eyelid margin

22. What diagnostic test is used to confirm the presence of entropion? *(608)*
    1. Amsler grid
    2. Snellen examination
    3. Ophthalmologic examination
    4. Pneumatic retinopexy

23. What type of visual distortion is associated with diabetic retinopathy? *(612)*
    1. Tunnel vision that worsens in low lighting
    2. Loss of visual acuity accompanied by "floaters"
    3. Sudden onset of peripheral vision loss and eye discomfort
    4. Difficulty distinguishing colors

24. A 65-year-old patient reports visual deficits, including disturbances in color vision and visual clarity, and a darkened area in the center of vision. What medical diagnosis does the nurse anticipate will be made? *(613)*
    1. Macular degeneration
    2. Glaucoma
    3. Herpetic keratitis
    4. Cataracts

25. Tonometry is used in the diagnosis of which condition? *(616)*
    1. Corneal abrasions
    2. Blepharitis
    3. Glaucoma
    4. Retinal detachment

26. The patient has been diagnosed with a visual disorder. Contact lenses have been prescribed. Which statement indicates the need for further instruction? *(604)*
    1. "Photophobia, dryness, burning, or tearing are expected symptoms."
    2. "I will use proper lens care solutions and a clean lens case."
    3. "I will need to be careful not to mix up my left and right lenses."
    4. "Washing and drying my hands before handling my lenses are essential."

27. Following cataract surgery, which activity is the ophthalmologist **most** likely to discourage? *(610)*
    1. Going to the movies
    2. Lifting a grandchild
    3. Walking on a sunny day
    4. Sleeping with a spouse

28. Based on research, supplemental zinc, beta-carotene, vitamins C and E, and a diet rich in fruits and dark-green leafy vegetables would be recommended for which eye disorder? *(612)*
    1. Age-related macular degeneration
    2. Senile cataracts
    3. Retinal detachment
    4. Glaucoma

29. A patient reports seeing flashing lights and floaters and a dark area in the outer peripheral vision. What is the **most** important question to ask for suspicion of retinal detachment? *(614)*
    1. "Are you having severe pain in the affected eye?"
    2. "Is the darkened area getting progressively larger?"
    3. "Do you have type 1 diabetes mellitus?"
    4. "Do you have a family history of eye problems?"

30. What are the current recommendations for ophthalmologic examinations? **Select all that apply.** *(618)*
    1. People between 40 and 64 years of age need examination every 2-4 years.
    2. People who wear contact lenses should have examinations every 6 months.
    3. African Americans in every age group should have more frequent examinations.
    4. People 65 years of age or older should be examined every 1-2 years.
    5. People with diabetes mellitus should have more frequent examinations.

31. The nurse's neighbor is trying to remove an eyelash from her eye. The nurse would intervene if the neighbor used which method? *(620)*
    1. Flushed the eye gently with tap water
    2. Tried blinking and crying to stimulate tears
    3. Used a clean cotton-tipped swab to wipe the cornea
    4. Used a sterile pad to wipe the corner of the eye

32. The nurse is on a camping trip and one of the campers gets poked in the eye with a stick. The end of the stick is protruding from the eye. What should the nurse do **first**? *(620)*
    1. Gently remove the stick and then flush the eye with water.
    2. Cover the injured eye with a paper cup and patch the uninjured eye.
    3. Have the camper sit quietly in the car and drive him to the hospital.
    4. Remain calm and control the bleeding with direct pressure.

33. What problem will the patient have if there is damage to the fine hair cell receptors in the organ of Corti? *(624)*
    1. Difficulty with balance
    2. Overproduction of cerumen
    3. Loss of hearing
    4. Blurred distance vision

34. The nurse overhears a nursing student giving advice to a patient to "get a hearing aid." What is the **best** response that the nurse could give to the student and the patient? *(626, 627)*
    1. "Let's focus on nursing interventions that we can use today; for example, face each other and speak clearly."
    2. "The care, maintenance, and usage of a hearing aid can be complex, so we should first talk about those issues."
    3. "This is a good suggestion. We will make you an appointment with your health care provider."
    4. "The type of hearing loss must first be determined because the device won't work for all types of hearing loss."

35. Which patient is likely to be the **best** candidate for a hearing aid? *(626)*
    1. Patient has congenital hearing loss secondary to oxygen deprivation at birth.
    2. Patient has conductive hearing loss due to stenosis of the external auditory canal.
    3. Patient has functional hearing loss after being trapped in a cave for several hours.
    4. Patient has central hearing loss secondary to a cerebrovascular accident (stroke).

36. The health care provider informs the nurse that the patient had an abnormal Romberg test. Which safety precaution will the nurse initiate? *(626)*
    1. Make sure the room has adequate natural lighting.
    2. Do a physical demonstration of how to use the call light.
    3. Announce self to avoid suddenly startling the patient.
    4. Assist the patient to stand and get balance before walking.

37. The nurse's toddler received a prescription for antibiotics to treat acute otitis media. The antibiotics and acetaminophen where given as recommended, but the toddler is still crying with pain. What should the nurse try **first**? *(629)*
    1. Have the toddler swallow cool fluids.
    2. Place a warm compress over the affected ear.
    3. Use distraction until the acetaminophen works.
    4. Call the provider and ask for a sedative prescription.

38. What is an **early** indicator of acute otitis media? *(629)*
    1. Patient reports ear pain and is pulling on the pinna.
    2. Patient reports partial hearing loss.
    3. There is yellow discharge with a pungent odor.
    4. Patient reports sensation of blockage in ear canal.

39. During the night, which strategy for environmental control is **best** to help the patient with tinnitus? *(635)*
    1. Have the patient lie very still.
    2. Play soft background music.
    3. Keep the room dark and quiet.
    4. Turn on the television.

40. The nurse is reviewing the patient's medication list and sees the patient takes meclizine. What instructions should be given to the unlicensed assistive personnel (UAP)? *(637)*
    1. Face the patient directly when speaking to him.
    2. Assist the patient to ambulate because he gets dizzy.
    3. Keep the head of the bed elevated at least 30 degrees.
    4. Assist the patient to clean his eyes with a clean washcloth.

41. Which intervention applies to positioning the patient after a stapedectomy? *(637)*
    1. Keep the operative side facing upward.
    2. Elevate the head of the bed to at least 90 degrees.
    3. Turn, cough, and deep-breathe every 2 hours.
    4. Use a neck brace for the first 2 hours.

42. If there is a disturbance in proprioception, which function will the patient have difficulty performing? *(638)*
    1. Walking up the stairs
    2. Understanding informed consent
    3. Reading prescription labels
    4. Listening to the provider's instructions

CRITICAL THINKING ACTIVITIES

Activity 1

43. An 18-year-old patient has just returned from surgery for the enucleation of his right eye after injuries suffered in an accident. *(621)*

    a. Discuss the nursing interventions that will be required over the next 24 hours. _____

    _____

    _____

    _____

b. What findings are indicative of complications and warrant an immediate report to the health care provider?

_____

_____

c. The patient expresses concerns about his appearance. How will the nurse address his concerns?

_____

_____

Activity 2

44. A 20-year-old patient reports worsening ear pain. After completing his history, it is determined he recently had an ear infection and he failed to take the full course of prescribed medications. His other signs and symptoms include fever, headache, malaise, and purulent exudate. *(632, 633)*

a. What should the nurse anticipate the patient's medical diagnosis will be? _____

_____

b. How did this condition occur? _____

_____

_____

c. Discuss the treatment and the prognosis for this condition. _____

_____

_____

_____

_____

Activity 3

45. The patient had vitrectomy surgery of the right eye. List the appropriate nursing interventions for this patient. *(622)*

_____

_____

_____

_____

_____

_____

_____

Activity 4

46. Refer to Box 13.2 and identify behaviors that you have noticed for someone who may be demonstrating hearing loss. Has that person admitted that he or she has hearing loss? *(625)*

_____

_____

_____

_____

Activity 5

47. If you were to suddenly lose your vision or hearing, how would the loss affect your current lifestyle and future plans? *(639)*

_____

_____

_____

_____

_____

_____

_____

_____

Student Name_____ Date_____

<table>
<tr><td rowspan="2">Care of the Patient With a
Neurologic Disorder</td><td>chapter</td></tr>
<tr><td>14</td></tr>
</table>

Answer Key: Textbook page references are provided as a guide for answering these questions. A complete Answer Key is provided in your Additional Learning Resources on Evolve.

FIGURE LABELING

1. Directions: Label the parts of the brain on the figure below. *(646)*

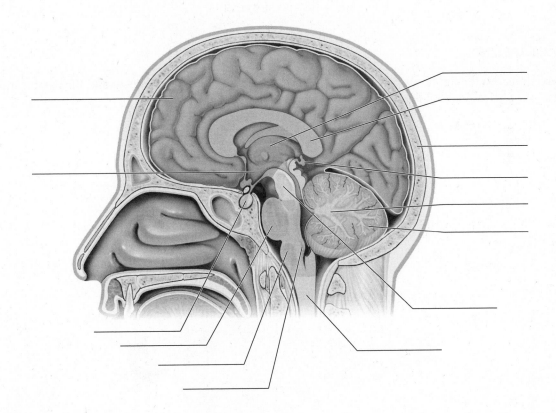

MATCHING

Directions: Match the cranial nerves to their functions. Indicate your answers in the spaces provided. (648)

Cranial Nerve

_____ 2. I—olfactory

_____ 3. II—optic

_____ 4. III—oculomotor

_____ 5. IV—trochlear

_____ 6. VI—abducens

_____ 7. VII—facial

_____ 8. VIII—acoustic (vestibulocochlear)

_____ 9. IX—glossopharyngeal

_____ 10. X—vagus

_____ 11. XI—spinal accessory

_____ 12. XII—hypoglossal

Functions

a. Eye movements, extraocular muscles, pupillary control (pupillary constriction)

b. Hearing; sense of balance (equilibrium)

c. Down and inward movement of eye

d. Shoulder movements (trapezius muscle) and turning movements of head (sternocleidomastoid muscles)

e. Sense of smell

f. Vision

g. Sense of taste on anterior two-thirds of tongue; contraction of muscles of facial expression

h. Sensations of throat, taste, swallowing movements, gag reflex, taste on posterior one-third of tongue, secretion of saliva

i. Lateral movement of eye

j. Sensations of throat, larynx, and thoracic and abdominal organs; swallowing; voice production; slowing of heartbeat; acceleration of peristalsis

k. Tongue movements

FIGURE LABELING

13. Directions: On the figures below, identify decorticate and decerebrate responses and the flexion and extension characteristics of the upper and lower extremities. *(661)*

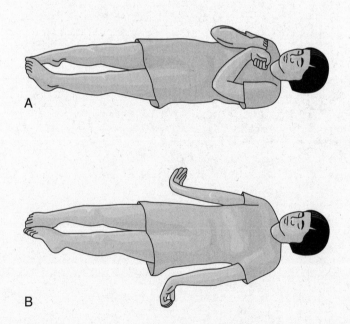

WORD SCRAMBLE

Levels of Consciousness

Directions: Unscramble the letters to reveal the correct spelling of terms related to level of consciousness and then match them to the correct definition or description. (651)

Scrambled Term	Unscrambled Term	Definition or Characteristic
14. treal		
15. orientdisation		
16. porstu		
17. tosecomasemi		
18. esotamoc		

Description

a. Responds to verbal commands with moaning or groaning, if at all; seems unaware of surroundings
b. Is in impaired state of consciousness characterized by obtundation and stupor, from which a patient can be aroused only by energetic stimulation
c. Unable to respond to painful stimuli; cornea and pupillary reflexes are absent; cannot swallow or cough; is incontinent of urine and feces; electroencephalogram pattern demonstrates decreased or absent neuronal activity
d. Unable to follow simple commands; thinking slowed; inattentive; flat affect
e. Responds appropriately to auditory, tactile, and visual stimuli

MULTIPLE CHOICE

Directions: Select the best answer(s) for each of the following questions.

19. In Parkinson's disease, which neurotransmitter is decreased and therefore is a target of medication therapy? *(673)*
    1. Acetylcholine
    2. Norepinephrine
    3. Dopamine
    4. Serotonin

20. In working with patients who have neurologic conditions that affect language function, which patient represents the **greatest** challenge to achieve communication? *(653)*
    1. Patient has anomic aphasia that developed after removal of brain tumor.
    2. Patient has global aphasia due to progressive Alzheimer's disease.
    3. Patient has motor aphasia secondary to head injury.
    4. Patient has receptive aphasia residual to a stroke.

21. Which behavior(s) would be considered normal neurologic changes related to aging? **Select all that apply.** *(650)*
    1. Drives slower to compensate for slowed reaction time
    2. Demonstrates slight tremor while holding teacup when tired
    3. Takes a foreign language class, but can't keep up with classmates
    4. Does needlework, but has more trouble with fine, small stitches
    5. Rearranges items on countertop, but action serves no purpose
    6. Frequently misplaces keys or eyeglasses, but can usually find them

22. The nurse is assessing the "fund of knowledge" component of the patient's awareness. Which question would the nurse use to assess this component? *(651)*
    1. "What month is it? And what day of the week is it today?"
    2. "What did you have for dinner last night?"
    3. "If you had $3.00 and gave me half, what would you have?"
    4. "Who was the first president of the United States?"

23. The nurse is assessing a patient who had a serious head injury. During the assessment, the patient spontaneously opens his eyes; is oriented to person, place, and time; and can follow the nurse's commands. How would the nurse document his Glasgow coma score (GCS)? *(651)*
    1. GCS within normal limits
    2. GCS insufficient
    3. GCS 3
    4. GCS 15

24. The nurse is using the FOUR Score coma scale to assess a patient who suffered a stroke. Which assessment is an integral part of this scale? *(651)*
    1. Checking the blood pressure and pulse
    2. Checking orientation to person, place, and time
    3. Assessing the respiratory rate and pattern
    4. Evaluating the ability to make good judgments

25. The nurse hears in report that the patient has motor aphasia. Which intervention will the nurse plan to use when communicating with this patient? *(652)*
    1. Talk slower, be patient, and enunciate very clearly.
    2. Face the patient so that he can watch the lips move.
    3. Obtain a set of picture cards and encourage gestures.
    4. Be kind and caring, but limit verbal communication.

26. The nurse is checking the gag reflex prior to giving liquids to a patient who had a bronchoscopy earlier in the day. Which cranial nerves is the nurse testing? *(648)*
    1. Optic and oculomotor
    2. Abducens and trochlear
    3. Trigeminal and facial
    4. Glossopharyngeal and vagus

27. The nurse is caring for a patient who has unilateral neglect that includes the nondominant hand. For which task is the patient **most** likely to require assistance? *(653)*
    1. Putting on her blouse
    2. Holding a drinking glass
    3. Using the remote control
    4. Writing a letter

28. The patient is scheduled to return from having a lumbar puncture. What instructions will the nurse give to the unlicensed assistive personnel (UAP) about the care of this patient? *(654)*
    1. Help the patient ambulate in the halls.
    2. Keep the head of the bed at 30 degrees.
    3. Withhold fluids for several hours.
    4. Report any complaints of numbness or tingling.

29. The nurse is caring for a patient who had cerebral angiogram and the vascular system was accessed through the carotid artery. In the immediate postprocedure assessment, what is the **priority**? *(656)*
    1. Watching for infection at the puncture site
    2. Assessing for reaction to contrast media
    3. Observing for respiratory difficulties
    4. Assessing for nausea and vomiting

30. A 35-year-old man who suffers from tension headaches requests opioid medications for the debilitating pain. Why is the health care provider unlikely to grant the patient's request? *(658)*
    1. Opioids are avoided because of the risk of abuse.
    2. Tension headache pain does not warrant opioid use.
    3. Pain receptor sites will not respond to opioids.
    4. Tension headaches are controlled by reducing stress.

31. Which food may cause or worsen a migraine headache? *(657)*
    1. Italian food
    2. Apples
    3. Dairy products
    4. Ripened cheese

32. In caring for a patient with a headache, which instruction will the nurse give to the UAP? *(658)*
    1. Assist the patient to turn every 2 hours.
    2. Keep the room quiet and dark.
    3. Refresh warm compress as needed.
    4. Withhold fluids because of nausea.

33. The nurse is reviewing the medication list for a patient who is diabetic and sees that gabapentin is prescribed. Which pain assessment will the nurse make? *(659)*
    1. Low back pain with movement
    2. Dull or throbbing headache
    3. Burning or tingling in lower legs
    4. Stiffness of joints in the morning

34. What is an **early** sign of increased intracranial pressure? *(661)*
    1. Change in level of consciousness
    2. Decreased or abnormal respirations
    3. Increased systolic blood pressure
    4. Increased or widening pulse pressure

35. The night shift nurse has just finished giving report on four patients who have risk for increased intracranial pressure. The health care provider is aware of their status. Which patient will the oncoming nurse check **first**? *(661)*
    1. Patient had a brief episode of Cheyne-Stokes respirations.
    2. Patient reported double vision and difficulty concentrating.
    3. Patient seemed restless and disoriented.
    4. Patient had a headache with nausea and vomiting.

36. The nurse is checking the pupils of a patient who sustained a serious head injury. Which pupil response is the **first** and most subtle clue of increased intracranial pressure? *(661)*
    1. Pupil reacts, but is sluggish.
    2. Pupil is fixed and dilated.
    3. Pupil is dilated, but will slowly constrict.
    4. Pupil on affected side is larger.

37. Which patient is **best** demonstrating the use of intact sensory abilities to independently compensate for a sensory deficit? *(666)*
    1. Patient with agnosia needs help for activities of daily living.
    2. Patient with loss of proprioception uses a walker.
    3. Patient with diabetic neuropathy inspects feet every day.
    4. Patient with hearing deficit speaks very loudly to others.

38. The nurse is planning patient education for several patients. Which patient is the **best** candidate for a teaching session on weight shifting? *(664)*
    1. Patient with mild Alzheimer's has recently started wandering.
    2. Patient has Parkinson's and shows evidence of pill-rolling.
    3. Patient with paraplegia is transferring to a rehabilitation unit.
    4. Patient has unilateral neglect that is affecting the dominant side.

39. For a patient with hemiplegia, how does the staff use counterpositioning to protect the affected upper extremity? *(664)*
    1. Positions the upper extremity with shoulder pulled inward and elbow extended
    2. Places the shoulder and upper arm in abduction with elbow flexed and wrist dorsiflexed
    3. Places the patient recumbent with arm beside body, elbow straight, and palmar surface upwards
    4. Elevates the elbow and forearm on a pillow above the level of the heart with wrist flexed

40. The home health nurse is reviewing the patient's medication list and sees that the patient takes phenytoin. Which question is the nurse **most** likely to ask? *(669)*
    1. "When was the last time you had a seizure?"
    2. "Has the medication controlled your headaches?"
    3. "When did you first start taking medication for Parkinson's?"
    4. "Has the medication helped to reduce the spasms?"

41. Which measures should be implemented for a patient experiencing increased intracranial pressure? **Select all that apply.** *(663)*
    1. Restrict fluid intake.
    2. Place head in flexed position.
    3. Avoid flexion of the hips.
    4. Administer enemas as needed.
    5. Administer oxygen.

42. The patient has residual hemiplegia following a stroke. Which instructions will the nurse give to the UAP? *(664)*
    1. Assist the patient to ambulate to the bathroom.
    2. Put the affected arm through range of motion.
    3. Place in a prone position if the patient can tolerate it.
    4. Use pillows to keep the upper arm in adduction.

43. The nurse hears in report that the 33-year-old patient with multiple sclerosis (MS) is withdrawn, depressed, and emotionally labile. The nurse knows that emotional changes are part of the disease. What other aspect(s) of the disease are likely to be contributing to the patient's emotional state? **Select all that apply.** *(671)*
    1. Exacerbations and remissions are continuous; deterioration progresses.
    2. The symptoms are vague, insidious, and widely distributed.
    3. No specific treatments exist, although many treatments have been tried.
    4. Multiple body systems are affected, and function is lost in every area.
    5. Earlier diagnosis and intervention could have stopped the deterioration.

44. A resident with Parkinson's disease lives at a long-term care facility. The patient has a flat facial expression, hand tremors, and bradykinesia. Which instruction will the nurse give to the UAP to address the bradykinesia? *(673)*
    1. He has a shuffling gait and needs assistance to prevent bumping into objects.
    2. He has trouble bending to tie his shoes because of muscle soreness and aches.
    3. He has trouble using a fork and knife because of loss of fine motor control.
    4. He has resistance to motion, so he may seem stiff when you put on his shirt.

45. The health care provider tells that nurse that during hospitalization, the older patient is going to be on drug holiday from all medications that are normally prescribed for his Parkinson's disease. What is the **priority** problem related to the temporary cessation of the medications? *(675)*
    1. Aspiration
    2. Constipation
    3. Tremors
    4. Postural hypotension

46. What is an **early** subjective symptom that the patient may report that would be characteristic of myasthenia gravis? *(681)*
    1. Muscle weakness in the extremities
    2. Eyelid drooping and double vision
    3. Trouble swallowing
    4. Weak, nasal-sounding voice

47. What is the **priority** assessment for a patient with a severe exacerbation of myasthenia gravis? *(683)*
    1. Assess for ocular signs/symptoms including ptosis and diplopia.
    2. Auscultate bowel sounds and assess bowel and bladder continence.
    3. Assess ability to ambulate, sustain a sitting position, and raise arms.
    4. Auscultate lungs, assess respiratory effort and ability to cough up secretions.

48. What is the single **most** important modifiable risk factor for stroke? *(684)*
    1. Cigarette smoking
    2. Sedentary lifestyle
    3. Hypertension
    4. Obesity

49. The patient who had a stroke exhibits dysphagia. Which intervention will the nurse use? *(689)*
    1. Mix solid and liquid foods together to facilitate swallowing.
    2. Assist the patient to drink water after every bite of food.
    3. Offer the patient a drinking straw or a covered plastic cup.
    4. Check mouth on the affected side for accumulation of food.

50. The patient comes to the clinic and is exhibiting stroke symptoms. The health care provider believes that the patient is a possible candidate for thrombolytic therapy. What are the **most** important actions for the clinic staff to perform? *(687)*
    1. Rapid triage and transport to a stroke center
    2. Draw blood for coagulation tests and establish IV
    3. Obtain a CT or MRI to rule out hemorrhagic stroke
    4. Explain the risks and benefits of therapy to the patient

51. In caring for a patient with trigeminal neural-
gia, what instructions would the nurse give
to the UAP about assisting with hygiene and
meals? *(690)*
    1. Use gentle touch when assisting with shav-
ing.
    2. Encourage the patient to drink cold liq-
uids.
    3. Allow the patient to do his own care if he
prefers.
    4. Offer to cut the patient's food into bite-
sized pieces.

52. A patient who is diagnosed with Bell's palsy
will need to know how to use which device?
(691)
    1. Eating utensil with a universal cuff
    2. Eyeshield to be applied at night
    3. Footboard for the end of the bed
    4. A volar wrist splint for extension

53. In caring for a patient who is diagnosed with
Guillain-Barré syndrome, what is the **priority**
assessment? *(692)*
    1. Motion and sensation in the legs
    2. Respiratory depth and pattern
    3. Mental status and level of consciousness
    4. Loss of bowel and bladder control

54. The nurse is caring for a patient who is diagnosed with bacterial meningitis. For this
patient, what is the rationale for keeping the
room quiet and dark? *(693)*
    1. Light and noise increase the subjective ex-
perience of pain.
    2. Patient needs extra rest and sleep to facili-
tate recovery.
    3. Any increased sensory stimulation may
cause a seizure.
    4. Critically ill patients do better in quiet en-
vironments.

55. What is considered a prominent **early** sign of a
brain tumor? *(696)*
    1. Speech impairment
    2. Morning headache
    3. Change in personality
    4. Memory loss

56. A young man who sustained a serious head
injury several years ago is a resident in a long-
term care facility. After the injury, he demon-
strated intermittent poor judgment and occasional physical aggression. Today, he is trying
to leave the facility. What should the nurse do
first? *(698)*
    1. Speak calmly and redirect him to another
activity.
    2. Obtain a prescription for an antianxiety
medication.
    3. Allow him to wander around but keep an
eye on him.
    4. Instruct a UAP to perform one-to-one ob-
servation.

57. The UAP tells the nurse that a patient with a
spinal cord injury has a systolic blood pressure of 190/100 mm Hg. The nurse observes
that the patient is diaphoretic, restless, and has
"gooseflesh" and a headache. What should the
nurse do **first**? *(701)*
    1. Recheck the blood pressure.
    2. Check the bladder for distention.
    3. Check the rectum for impaction.
    4. Put the patient in a sitting position.

58. For patients with spinal cord injuries, which
patient is **most** likely to achieve the rehabilitation potential of "Completely independent
ambulation with short leg braces and canes; inability to stand for long periods." *(700)*
    1. Patient has a level of injury at C8 sustained
in a diving accident.
    2. Patient has a level of injury at T12 related
to an occupational incident.
    3. Patient has a level of injury at L1 second-
ary to a gunshot wound.
    4. Patient has a level of injury at L4 sustained
in a motorcycle accident.

CRITICAL THINKING ACTIVITIES

Activity 1

59. The school nurse is accompanying a group of children on a field trip. One of children suddenly reports feeling odd and then sits down on the ground. As the nurse eases her to a supine position, the child demonstrates tonic-clonic jerking movements of the body. The nurse notes secretions and drooling from the child's mouth and the lips are slightly cyanotic. The child is unable to respond to her name and her eyes are rolled back and upwards. *(670)*

   a. Describe what the nurse should do. _____

   _____

   _____

   b. What information should the nurse record and report to the health care provider? _____

   _____

   _____

Activity 2

60. A 58-year-old man reports he experienced numbness in his right leg, a loss of sensation in his right arm, and an inability to speak; the entire event lasted only about 15 minutes. *(685)*

   a. What condition/disorder has the patient experienced? _____

   b. Since the duration of this event was short, is it of any long-term significance? Why or why not?

   _____

   _____

   _____

   c. What is the most frequently prescribed antiplatelet agent for this condition? _____

   _____

Activity 3

61. a. It is likely that you know or will know someone who has Alzheimer's disease. What are the warning signs? *(679)*

   _____

   _____

   _____

   _____

b. Discuss the effect that Alzheimer's disease has on family and society. *(680)* _____

_____

_____

_____

_____

c. What can you teach your patients to do that will help prevent Alzheimer's disease? *(679)* _____

_____

_____

_____

_____

Care of the Patient With an Immune Disorder

Answer Key: Textbook page references are provided as a guide for answering these questions. A complete Answer Key is provided in your Additional Learning Resources on Evolve.

FIGURE LABELING

1. Directions: Label the figure below with the correct names of the organs of the immune system. *(710)*

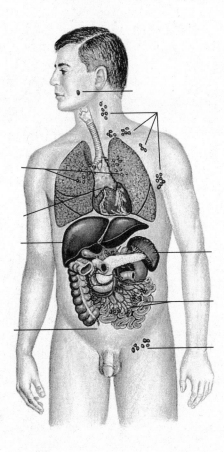

SHORT ANSWER

Directions: Using your own words, answer each question in the space provided.

2. What are the three main functions of the immune system? *(708)*

    a. _____

    b. _____

    c. _____

3. What are the four Rs of the immune response? *(712)*

    a. _____

    b. _____

    c. _____

    d. _____

4. Identify the five factors influencing hypersensitivity. *(714)*

    a. _____

    b. _____

    c. _____

    d. _____

    e. _____

5. List 14 items in the health care environment that could contain latex. *(718)* _____

    _____

    _____

MULTIPLE CHOICE

Directions: Select the best answer(s) for each of the following questions.

6. Which nursing action **best** supports the patient's innate immunity? *(709)*
    1. Encourages the patient to complete full course of prescribed antibiotics
    2. Advises older patient to get an annual influenza vaccination
    3. Assists new mother who is learning to breastfeed her baby
    4. Assesses the skin of a patient who is at risk for a pressure injury

7. Which surgical procedure creates lifetime immunocompromise and vulnerability to infection? *(720)*
    1. Thyroidectomy
    2. Splenectomy
    3. Appendectomy
    4. Cholecystectomy

8. One of the residents in a long-term care facility has uncharacteristic lethargy and disorientation. The nurse recognizes that these could be early signs of infection. What would the nurse do **first**? *(713)*
    1. Obtain a prescription for white blood cell count.
    2. Obtain a urine specimen.
    3. Auscultate the breath sounds.
    4. Check the resident's temperature.

9. Which person needs to be advised to get the human papilloma virus vaccination? *(713)*
   1. 21-year-old sexually active male who has never been previously vaccinated
   2. 3-month-old who needs a well-baby physical and routine vaccination
   3. 73-year-old with chronic health problems who lives in a long-term care facility
   4. 54-year-old who is undergoing renal dialysis and is on the transplant list

10. Based on the National Institute for Occupational Safety and Health (NIOSH) recommendations for preventing allergic reactions to latex in the workplace, what instructions would the nurse give to the unlicensed assistive personnel (UAP)? *(718)*
    1. Avoid latex exposures and know the signs/symptoms of allergic response.
    2. Ask every patient about latex allergies before donning gloves.
    3. Do not use latex gloves unless there is visible evidence of blood and body fluid.
    4. Wash hands with a mild soap and dry thoroughly after removing latex gloves.

11. The home health patient thinks he has food allergies because he has diarrhea after eating certain foods. What would the nurse suggest **first**? *(715)*
    1. See the health care provider for possible desensitization therapy.
    2. Keep a weekly food diary with a description of any untoward reactions.
    3. Eliminate soy, eggs, and strawberries because of chance for anaphylaxis.
    4. Eat a bland diet and add a new food every week to see if there is a reaction.

12. In caring for an older adult, what instructions would the nurse give to the UAP that address changes related to aging of the immune system? **Select all that apply.** *(713)*
    1. Promptly assist with toileting to prevent urinary stasis.
    2. Increase fluids (unless contraindicated) to thin secretions.
    3. Apply a thin layer of lotion after bathing to prevent dry skin.
    4. Teach coughing and deep breathing as needed.
    5. Perform scrupulous hand hygiene and don clean gloves.
    6. Offer frequent oral hygiene because of decreased saliva production.

13. What is the theory behind progressively increasing the doses of the allergens during perennial immunotherapy? *(713)*
    1. Inhibits the release of leukotrienes and reduces allergic symptoms
    2. Allows the individual to build up a tolerance without having symptoms
    3. Competes with histamine by attaching to the cell surface receptors
    4. Inhibits further release of chemical mediators from mast cells

14. If medications are administered in error to a patient who is hypersensitive, which route will produce the **most** rapid allergic reaction? *(714)*
    1. Oral
    2. Transdermal
    3. Intravenous
    4. Topical

15. The nurse and a friend are ordering lunch. The friend takes 50 mg of diphenhydramine and then orders oysters, saying, "I'm allergic to oysters, but I just love them, so I take medication." What should the nurse say? *(714)*
    1. "Do you have your cell phone, so we can call 911?"
    2. "Every time you eat oysters, the reaction will get worse."
    3. "You are an adult and you can make your own choices."
    4. "If I have to resuscitate you, I am not going to be happy."

16. The clinic nurse is trying to do an environmental assessment for an older patient who is having continuous allergic reactions, but the patient vaguely rambles on about pets, dust, a broken vacuum cleaner, and mold. What is the **best** intervention to use for this patient? *(714)*
    1. Use simplified, focused yes-or-no questions.
    2. Make an environmental checklist for the patient.
    3. Obtain information from a close relative.
    4. Obtain an order for a home health nurse visit.

17. Within 15 minutes of initiating a blood transfusion, the patient reports shortness of breath, chills, and urticaria. After stopping the transfusion and notifying the health care provider, which laboratory test must be completed? *(719)*
    1. Urinalysis
    2. Electrolytes
    3. Platelet count
    4. White blood cell count

18. What is the physiologic explanation for the suppressed humoral immune response in older adults? *(720)*
    1. Degeneration of the spleen
    2. Decreased production of white blood cells
    3. Reduction in effectiveness of white blood cells
    4. Decreased immunoglobulin levels

19. During plasmapheresis, the plasma may be replaced with what? **Select all that apply.** *(721)*
    1. Normal saline
    2. Lactated Ringer's solution
    3. Albumin
    4. 10% dextrose
    5. Fresh-frozen plasma
    6. Dextrose 5% and half normal saline

20. The nurse gives a patient his immunotherapy injection and immediately he demonstrates wheezes, impaired breathing, and hypotension. The nurse initiates the anaphylaxis protocol. What is the nurse's **first** action? *(717)*
    1. Establish an IV to administer 1:10,000 epinephrine hydrochloride.
    2. Administer 1:1000 epinephrine hydrochloride subcutaneously.
    3. Prepare the equipment and assist the provider to intubate the patient.
    4. Administer a 50-mg oral dose of diphenhydramine.

21. What are examples of passive immunity? **Select all that apply.** *(711)*
    1. Mother breastfeeds her baby
    2. Antivenom given after a snakebite
    3. Immunoglobulin administered postexposure
    4. Child gets hepatitis B vaccine
    5. Patient reports having measles during childhood

22. In caring for a patient who recently had an organ transplant, which instructions would the nurse give to the UAP to protect this immunosuppressed patient? *(719)*
    1. The most dangerous period is 7-10 days after the transplant.
    2. Remind visitors to check at the nurses' station before entering.
    3. If you are pregnant, the patient's chemotherapy may harm the baby.
    4. If you have a cough or skin infection, don a mask and gown.

23. The nurse is caring for a patient who underwent plasmapheresis. What is the **most** important assessment to make after the procedure? *(721)*
    1. Monitor intake and output.
    2. Check blood pressure.
    3. Assess mental status.
    4. Evaluate pain.

CRITICAL THINKING ACTIVITIES

Activity 1

24. A 22-year-old patient has just completed allergy testing. Her health care provider has prescribed a regimen of weekly allergy shots.

    a. What special precautions should be taken after the injection? *(713)* _____

    _____

    _____

b. What teaching should be provided for a patient who is receiving allergy shots at home? *(716)*

_____

_____

_____

c. After administering the shots at home for more than a month, the patient calls and reports she has been ill and unable to take the medications for the past 2 weeks. How should the nurse advise the patient? *(714)*

_____

_____

Activity 2

25. A 67-year-old patient voices concern about his health status. He reports he never used to "get sick," but now has been hospitalized three times in the last year with a variety of illnesses. *(713)*

a. Discuss how aging affects the immune system. _____

_____

_____

_____

b. For an older patient, what would the nurse recommend to decrease risk for infection? _____

_____

_____

_____

Activity 3

26. Design actual questions that the nurse could use to take a detailed history about a rash to help the health care provider diagnose the patient's allergies. Include: (1) onset, nature, and progression of signs and symptoms; (2) aggravating and alleviating factors; (3) frequency and duration of signs and symptoms; and (4) environmental, household, and occupational factors. *(714)*

_____

_____

_____

_____

_____

_____

_____

Care of the Patient With HIV/AIDS

Answer Key: Textbook page references are provided as a guide for answering these questions. A complete Answer Key is provided in your Additional Learning Resources on Evolve.

SHORT ANSWER

Directions: Using your own words, answer each question in the space provided.

1. List at least four common opportunistic diseases associated with HIV. *(739)*_____

_____

_____

_____

_____

2. List at least four barriers to adherence with HIV treatment recommendations. *(744)* _____

_____

_____

_____

_____

3. List three questions that the nurse should ask when talking to new patients to evaluate risk assessment specific to HIV and sexually transmitted infections, as well as blood-borne diseases. *(747)*

_____

_____

_____

MULTIPLE CHOICE

Directions: Select the best answer(s) for each of the following questions.

4. HIV is transmitted from human to human through infected body fluids. Which body fluids are considered vehicles of transmission? **Select all that apply.** *(755)*
   1. Blood
   2. Semen
   3. Cervicovaginal secretions
   4. Rectal secretions
   5. Urine
   6. Saliva

5. The nurse is teaching a patient living with HIV and her family about transmission of HIV. Which actions can the family and patient feel reassured are safe? **Select all that apply.** *(727)*
   1. Hugging
   2. Shaking hands
   3. Breastfeeding the baby
   4. Sharing a computer keyboard
   5. Sharing food and utensils
   6. Petting and playing with the family dog

6. The nurse is on a committee to plan a series of educational programs for prevention of HIV. For the first program, the committee decides to focus on the most common mode of transmission and the people at greatest risk. Which group will be the **first** target audience? *(727)*
   1. Receptive partners of men who have sex with men
   2. Heterosexual women who have sex with infected partners
   3. People who inject illicit drugs and share needles with others
   4. Health care workers who have occupational exposure

7. Which behavior combined with viral load status creates the **highest** risk for contracting HIV? *(727)*
   1. Infected partner in mid-stage HIV performs insertive oral intercourse.
   2. Uninfected partner receives anal intercourse from infected partner in primary stage.
   3. Infected partner in mid-stage receives vaginal intercourse from uninfected partner.
   4. Uninfected partner performs insertive oral intercourse on infected partner in late stage.

8. What factors increase the risk of HIV for intravenous drug users? **Select all that apply.** *(756)*
   1. Poor nutritional status and poor hygiene
   2. Exchanges sexual activity for drugs
   3. Impaired judgment due to illicit drug use
   4. Less likely to use condoms during sex
   5. Has ready access to sterile equipment
   6. Shares cookers and other paraphernalia

9. Which health care worker has sustained the **greatest** risk for HIV after being exposed to body fluids from patients who are HIV-positive? *(757)*
   1. Deep puncture with a hollow-bore needle filled with blood from a patient's vein
   2. Splashed in the face with saliva and mucus during oral suctioning and hygiene
   3. Glove tears while cleaning the perianal area of a patient who has postpartum bleeding
   4. Patient vomits copious amounts of bloody fluid over the front of the worker's uniform

10. For a health care worker who must take postexposure antiviral therapy, which signs/symptoms suggest that the worker is developing the **most** likely adverse effect of the drug therapy? *(729)*
    1. Fatigue, activity intolerance, and a low red blood cell count
    2. Decreased urine output and elevated blood urea nitrogen
    3. Jaundice, malaise, and abnormal liver function tests
    4. Chest pain, arrhythmias, and elevated troponin levels

11. Perinatal or vertical transmission has been reduced by initiating which combination of interventions? *(729)*
    1. Breastfeeding, enhanced maternal nutrition, and voluntary HIV testing
    2. Bottle-feeding, antiretroviral therapy for HIV-infected mothers, and cesarean birth
    3. Early prenatal care, natural childbirth, and antiretroviral therapy for HIV-infected babies
    4. Inducing labor during mid-stage HIV, and giving zidovudine syrup to neonate at birth

12. For a CD$_4^+$ lymphocyte level of 200 cells/mm^3, which clinical manifestations are **most** likely to be observed? *(724)*
    1. Generally asymptomatic
    2. Mild flulike symptoms
    3. Opportunistic infections
    4. Fatal respiratory complications

13. What differentiates typical progressors from long-term nonprogressors and rapid progressors? *(725)*
    1. Their physiologic response to standard antiviral therapy
    2. The age of the patient (i.e., rapid progressors are usually older)
    3. The length of time between seroconversion and symptom onset
    4. The number and combination of risk factors at time of exposure

14. What is the **primary** concern for a patient who has acute retroviral syndrome? *(734)*
    1. Focus of care is palliative and life expectancy is approximately 3 years.
    2. Risk for opportunistic infections is increased and infections are less responsive to medication.
    3. Fever, night sweats, chronic diarrhea, headaches, and fatigue affect activities of daily living.
    4. Viral load and risk of transmission are extremely high, but symptoms are minor and mild.

15. The patient is advised to be tested for viral load 4-6 months after exposure. What is the clinical significance of having a lower viral set point at this stage? *(734)*
    1. Used to determine the risk for exposing partner to HIV
    2. Predicts minor transient respiratory or skin infections
    3. Helps to determine the type and timing of therapy
    4. Used as a predictor of long-term survival

16. A 32-year-old patient diagnosed with HIV reports she is looking into some alternative and complementary therapies to treat her disease. What is the **best** response? *(740)*
    1. "You should only rely on prescribed medications."
    2. "Those therapies can be costly and ineffective."
    3. "What kind of therapies are you considering?"
    4. "Let me know how they work for you."

17. While caring for a known HIV-positive patient in the emergency department, the nurse notices the phlebotomist preparing to draw blood. Which nursing action is correct? *(740)*
    1. Do nothing, because all patients should be treated with Standard Precautions.
    2. Pull the technician aside and inform him about the patient's HIV status.
    3. Flag the chart to let all health care professionals know the patient's status.
    4. Discreetly hand a second pair of gloves to the technician as a signal.

18. An HIV-positive patient voices concern about his recurring bouts of diarrhea because he is making every effort to follow the treatment plan. What factors contribute to the diarrhea? **Select all that apply.** *(748)*
    1. Side effects of the medications
    2. Infections of the gastrointestinal tract
    3. Damage to the intestinal villi
    4. Malabsorption in the intestinal tract
    5. Insufficient personal hygiene

19. A 34-year-old patient has recently been diagnosed with HIV-associated cognitive motor complex. Which assessment will the home health nurse initiate? *(751)*
    1. Presence of numbness or tingling in hands or feet
    2. Level of consciousness based on Glasgow coma scale
    3. Home safety assessment to identify obstacles in hallways
    4. Pain in the extremities when ambulating or bending

20. The nurse is talking to a 17-year-old sexually active adolescent who is reluctant to use condoms because "It just doesn't feel as good." Which barrier to prevention is the adolescent demonstrating? *(754)*
    1. Denial of risk
    2. Fear of alienation
    3. Lack of access
    4. Anxiety about sex

21. Which sexual activity would be considered the **safest**? *(755)*
    1. Mutual monogamy
    2. Mutual masturbation
    3. Vaginal sex with condom
    4. Serial monogamy

22. What is a common presenting condition for HIV-positive women? *(735)*
    1. Shingles
    2. Syphilis
    3. Vaginal candidiasis
    4. Weakness in extremities

23. Which breakfast tray offers the **best** selection of foods for a patient who has oral thrush? *(751)*
    1. Grapefruit, hash browns, and an egg
    2. Oatmeal, vanilla yogurt, and canned peaches
    3. Orange juice, whole-wheat toast and jam
    4. Breakfast burrito with egg, bacon, and salsa

24. Which instructions about hygiene would the nurse give to the unlicensed assistive personnel (UAP) in assisting the patient who is living with HIV? *(742)*
    1. Avoid washing any skin lesions.
    2. Check for areas of dependent edema.
    3. Add oil to tub bath if rash is present.
    4. Use a soft toothbrush and nonabrasive toothpaste.

25. The home health nurse is visiting a patient who has end-stage HIV disease. The patient's partner is the primary caregiver and other members of the family are also available to help. What is the **most** important goal of palliative care for this patient and family? *(744)*
    1. Make plans for long-term care or home health assistance.
    2. Ensure that family complies with medication therapy.
    3. Relieve suffering caused by pain or other symptoms.
    4. Assess for disenfranchised grief and use active listening.

CRITICAL THINKING ACTIVITIES

Activity 1

26. A nursing student has just been stuck by a needle while providing care for a patient whose lifestyle has placed him at high risk for HIV infection. After reporting to the clinic, she has questions. *(757)*

    a. What course of action should be taken initially? _____

    _____

    _____

    _____

    b. What patient-based factors will affect her level of susceptibility? _____

    _____

    _____

    _____

c.   Upon hearing the recommendation for her to begin prophylactic drug therapy, she asks to wait a few days before beginning the medication regimen. What is the best advice?

_____

_____

_____

_____

d.   After a discussion of the need to begin the medications as soon as possible, she asks for an explanation concerning the pros and cons of taking the drugs.

_____

_____

_____

e.   The student voices concerns about having contact with her husband and child. How will the nurse respond to her concerns?

_____

_____

_____

_____

Activity 2

27.   A commercial sex worker has used the clinic for treatment for sexually transmitted infections over the past 3 years, but has always declined testing for HIV. Recently, the worker started to come in for a variety of infections that never seemed to fully resolve. Several nurses and health care providers talked to this patient about HIV testing and the benefits of early detection, but the patient said she assumes a "don't know, don't tell" position and that she tries to get all of her customers to use condoms. Several months later, the worker is admitted to the hospital for treatment of opportunistic infection secondary to HIV disease. Discuss the legal and ethical dilemmas for the clinic staff. *(757)*

_____

_____

_____

_____

_____

_____

_____

_____

Activity 3

28. Think about your personal feelings and concerns about taking care of a patient with HIV or AIDS. If possible, interview a nurse (or a patient) who experienced the early days of the HIV epidemic. Compare your own personal feelings to those of people who experienced the early days of HIV disease. *(723-725, 784)*

_____

_____

_____

_____

_____

_____

_____

_____

_____

_____

Care of the Patient With Cancer

Answer Key: Textbook page references are provided as a guide for answering these questions. A complete Answer Key is provided in your Additional Learning Resources on Evolve.

MATCHING

Directions: Match the terms to the correct definition. Indicate your answers in the spaces provided.

Terms

_____ 1. benign *(767)*

_____ 2. carcinoma *(768)*

_____ 3. differentiated *(767)*

_____ 4. malignant *(767)*

_____ 5. metastasis *(767)*

_____ 6. neoplasm *(767)*

_____ 7. sarcoma *(768)*

Definition

a. Malignant tumors

b. Process by which tumor cells spread

c. Abnormal cell growth with a loss of normal role and function, and ability to spread to other body sites

d. Malignant tumors of connective tissues

e. Uncontrolled or abnormal growth of cells

f. Recognizable as being the same in size or shape as normal cells

g. Not recurrent or progressive; nonmalignant

SHORT ANSWER

8. What are four quality-of-life factors that affect cancer patients and their families? *(786)*

a. _____

b. _____

c. _____

d. _____

9. Name at least five common concerns voiced by cancer patients. *(786)*

a. _____

b. _____

c. _____

d. _____

e. _____

10. What are the leading primary cancer sites for men? *(761)*

   a. _____

   b. _____

   c. _____

   d. _____

11. What are the leading primary cancer sites for women? *(761)*

   a. _____

   b. _____

   c. _____

   d. _____

12. What are the eight warning signs of cancer? *(766)*

   a. _____

   b. _____

   c. _____

   d. _____

   e. _____

   f. _____

   g. _____

   h. _____

FIGURE LABELING

13. Directions: On the figure below, identify the four types of biopsy depicted. *(769)*

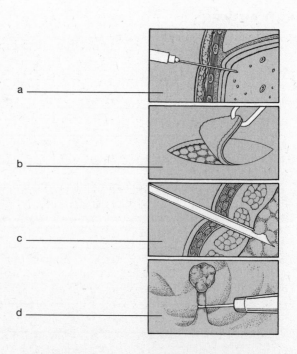

a _____

b _____

c _____

d _____

CLINICAL APPLICATION OF MATH

14. The American Cancer Society recommends adults engage in at least 150 minutes of moderate physical activity each week or 75 minutes of vigorous activity each week. *(767)*
    a. Patient A desires to exercise five times a week doing moderate physical exercise. How many minutes per day will the patient have to spend for each session? _____ min
    b. Patient B desires to exercise six times a week doing moderate physical exercise. How many minutes per day will the patient have to spend for each session? _____ min
    c. Patient C desires to exercise three times a week doing vigorous physical exercise. How many minutes per day will the patient have to spend for each session? _____ min
    d. Patient D desires to exercise seven times a week doing vigorous physical exercise. How many minutes per day will the patient have to spend for each session? _____ min

15. The nurse knows that a 5% weight loss places the patient at risk for malnutrition and the health care provider should be notified. If the patient weighs 140 pounds, how many pounds would be considered a 5% loss? _____ pounds *(785)*

16. The nutritionist tells the home health nurse that a 4.5 kg weight loss makes it difficult for the patient to maintain adequate nutritional status. The nurse closely monitors the patient's weight and nutritional intake. The patient weighed 123 lbs at the initial home health visit; today the patient weighs 118.5 lbs. How many kilograms has the patient lost? _____ kg *(785)*

TABLE ACTIVITY

17. Directions: Fill in the normal values in the table below. *(779)*

	Male	**Female**
Erythrocytes (RBCs)	million/mm³	million/mm³
Hemoglobin	g/dL	g/dL
Hematocrit	%	%

MULTIPLE CHOICE

Directions: Select the best answer(s) for each of the following questions.

18. Which person has the **greatest** risk for developing cancer? *(763)*
    1. Older white male who started smoking at age 14
    2. Middle-age obese white female with sedentary lifestyle
    3. Young African American woman who is a vegetarian
    4. Older Asian American male who drinks socially

19. Based on the incidence of cancer and the mortality rate, which group has the **greatest** need for improvements in cancer prevention, detection, and treatment outcomes? *(763)*
    1. Hispanic American females
    2. White American males
    3. Asian Americans
    4. African Americans

20. Which lunch tray contains the **best** selection of foods to reduce cancer risk? *(763)*
    1. Three-bean salad with cheddar cheese and saltine crackers
    2. Cottage cheese with tomatoes and melon ball salad
    3. Bacon, lettuce, and tomato on wheat toast with potato chips
    4. Grilled fish with white rice and pickled vegetables

21. What is the clinical significance for persons who have the *BRCA1* and *BRCA2* genes? *(764)*
    1. Increased incidence of lung cancer
    2. Increased incidence of leukemia
    3. Increased incidence of colon cancer
    4. Increased incidence of breast cancer

22. The nurse is volunteering at a local health fair and is talking with people about cancer prevention and screening recommendations. Which person should be referred for cancer risk assessment and genetic counseling? *(764)*
    1. Admits to a long history of smoking tobacco and marijuana
    2. History of multiple primary cancers in one family member
    3. Has an occupational history of exposure to heavy metals
    4. Has a recent change in bowel movements with occasional bleeding

23. What is a clinical manifestation of testicular cancer? *(765)*
    1. Erectile dysfunction
    2. Weak flow of urine
    3. An enlargement in either testicle
    4. Smooth consistency of testicles

24. Which person is the **most** likely candidate for low-dose helical CT for lung cancer screening? *(766)*
    1. 35-year-old male who never smoked, but is anxious because his father died of lung cancer
    2. 55-year-old male quit smoking 5 years ago and is in fairly good health with a 30 pack-year history
    3. 25-year-old female has smoked for 10 years and is unable to accomplish smoking cessation
    4. 69-year-old female smoked for several years during her early twenties, but is currently healthy

25. What instructions should be given to boys and men about self-examination of the testes? **Select all that apply.** *(765)*
    1. Should be done once a month.
    2. Feel for lumps or thickening.
    3. Check after a warm bath or shower.
    4. Self-examination should begin at puberty.
    5. Men older than 50 should stop self-examination.

26. Which dietary recommendation to decrease risk for cancer comes from the National Cancer Institute? *(763)*
    1. Eat four to five servings of lean protein each day.
    2. Eat at least two servings of yellow cheese each day.
    3. Add several types of beans to your diet every week.
    4. Eat at least five servings of fruit and vegetables each day.

27. The patient states that she knows vitamin C is an important nutrient in the prevention of cancer, but she really dislikes citrus fruits. What is the **best** alternative source that the nurse could suggest? *(763)*
    1. Taking a vitamin C supplement
    2. Trying citrus juice in place of fruit
    3. Eating strawberries or tomatoes
    4. Eating carrots or cauliflower

28. The nurse is talking to a 23-year-old woman about breast self-examination (BSE). What does the nurse tell the patient about timing and frequency of doing BSE? *(764)*
    1. Perform the examination monthly on the first day of your menses.
    2. Perform the examination on the first day of every month.
    3. Perform the examination if you notice a discharge from the nipple.
    4. Perform the examination 2-3 days after your period ends.

29. A prostate-specific antigen (PSA) test is usually recommended at age 50. Beginning at age 40, members of which ethnic group need to be advised to get the test? *(771)*
    1. Asian American
    2. African American
    3. Native American
    4. Hispanic American

30. According to clinical staging classification, which stage indicates the **most** extensive cancer with the poorest prognosis? *(768)*
    1. Stage 0
    2. Stage I
    3. Stage III
    4. Stage IV

31. According to the TNM classification system, which set of parameters suggests the **best** prognosis? *(768)*
    1. $T_0; N_0; M_0$
    2. $T_x; N_x; M_x$
    3. $T_{is}; N_1; M_1$
    4. $T_4; N_4; M_4$

32. The patient is having a radioisotope bone scan. He has had the radioactive material injected into his arm and the nurse encourages him to drink water for the next several hours. What is the purpose of encouraging fluids? *(770)*
    1. Radioisotope that is not picked up by the bone will be flushed through the kidneys.
    2. The radioactive material could be harmful to the kidneys if not diluted and voided.
    3. The fluid enhances the contrast media and facilitates visualization of tumor areas.
    4. Extra fluid thins secretions and improves the visualization of the lung fields.

33. The health care provider is considering magnetic resonance imaging (MRI) for a patient who might have a spinal tumor. Prior to the MRI, the nurse would notify the provider if the patient disclosed which information? *(770)*
    1. History of depression
    2. Family history of breast cancer
    3. History of hip fracture
    4. History of deep vein thrombosis

34. The health care provider informs the nurse that the patient may have metastasis to the bone. The provider requests that the nurse notify her immediately with the relevant results. Which test will the nurse be watching for? *(770)*
    1. Serum calcitonin
    2. Alkaline phosphatase
    3. Carcinoembryonic antigen
    4. CA-125

35. The patient has a positive guaiac test, but he tells the nurse that he may have not followed the dietary instructions correctly. Which food substance is **most** likely to cause a false positive? *(773)*
    1. A rare steak
    2. A double fudge sundae
    3. French fries with catsup
    4. Caffeinated soda

36. The nurse is present when the health care provider tells the patient that a combination of surgery, radiation, and chemotherapy are needed to treat his cancer. Afterwards, the patient angrily says, "I'm not going to spend my last days getting poked by that doctor. I'm leaving the hospital!" What should the nurse say? *(774)*
    1. "I respect your decision, but is there anything I can do to help?"
    2. "Don't be hasty, you have just had bad news; wait for a while."
    3. "Please don't leave. The doctor is just trying to help you."
    4. "You are upset; that's understandable. Let me call your doctor."

37. The unlicensed assistive personnel (UAP) is assigned to assist with hygiene for a patient who is currently undergoing external radiation over a large portion of the trunk. What instructions will the nurse give? *(775)*
    1. Gently clean the skin with a mild soap and flush with warm water.
    2. Do not put lotion, cream, or body powder over the marked areas.
    3. Help the patient take a shower, but use tepid water and a soft cloth.
    4. Shower according to usual procedure, but don't scrub the skin.

38. In caring for the patient who is being treated with internal radiation, what is the **most** important part of the nursing process for the nurse to prevent self-exposure? *(776)*
    1. Assessment
    2. Planning
    3. Implementation
    4. Evaluation

39. The UAP is assigned to assist a patient who is being treated with radioactive material in the vagina. What instructions should the nurse give? *(776)*
    1. Spend a maximum of 10 minutes to help with a bed bath from the waist up.
    2. Assist the patient with perineal care because vaginal discharge is likely.
    3. Help the patient ambulate to the shower if she is feeling well enough to walk.
    4. Turn the patient every 2 hours and remind her to do range-of-motion for her arms.

40. The patient is placed on neutropenic precautions for a neutrophil count of fewer than 1000/mm³. Which prescription would the nurse question? *(777)*
    1. Take vital signs every 4 hours.
    2. Report temperature greater than 100.4° F (38° C).
    3. Catheterize for urine specimen.
    4. Administer filgrastim.

41. Which intervention is the nurse **most** likely to use for a patient who has "chemo brain"? *(777)*
    1. Frequently orient the patient to person, place, and time.
    2. Perform the Glasgow coma scale at least once per shift.
    3. Help patient to establish routine and avoid multi-tasking.
    4. Instruct UAP to assist with most activities of daily living.

42. The patient has stomatitis secondary to chemotherapy. Which intervention will the nurse use? *(778)*
    1. Suggest that the patient suck hard candy or chew gum.
    2. Help the patient rinse with mouthwash every 2-4 hours.
    3. Use a sponge-tipped applicator to perform frequent mouth care.
    4. Suggest drinking warm soup, tea, or other hot liquids.

43. The patient is receiving epoetin alfa. Which laboratory finding indicates that the therapy is helping? *(779)*
    1. Normalization of the white cell count
    2. Improvement of the red cell count
    3. Increase in the platelet count
    4. Normalization of the electrolytes

44. Which observation would be consistent with a platelet count of fewer than 20,000/mm³? *(779)*
    1. Extreme fatigue
    2. Decreased urine output
    3. High fever
    4. Bleeding gums

45. While caring for a 23-year-old patient undergoing chemotherapy, the patient voices concerns about her hair loss. What information would the nurse give to the patient? *(779)*
    1. The loss of her hair will not be permanent.
    2. Hair loss will only affect facial areas.
    3. The hair just stops growing temporarily.
    4. When the hair grows back, it will be thicker.

46. During meal planning for a cancer patient, the patient reports that things have a "strange" taste, which is affecting her appetite. Which responses accurately pertain to her concern? **Select all that apply.** *(785)*
    1. This is a common occurrence and will get better after the treatment ends.
    2. Taste alteration is a permanent consequence associated with treatment.
    3. Onion and ham may help to improve the taste of vegetables.
    4. Lemon juice is successfully used to mask strange taste sensations.
    5. Eat anything that seems appealing, just try to maintain the caloric intake.

47. Which factors are shown to have an impact on how a patient will cope with a diagnosis of cancer? **Select all that apply.** *(786)*
    1. Age at the time of the diagnosis
    2. Availability of significant others
    3. Presence of symptoms
    4. Socioeconomic status
    5. Gender
    6. Ability to express feelings

48. The nurse is reviewing the patient's medication list and sees that the patient is taking ondansetron. What additional intervention will the nurse plan to use? *(780)*
    1. Minimize food odors or noxious smells.
    2. Help the patient dangle before walking.
    3. Check the pulse before giving the drug.
    4. Place a sign on the door to limit visitors.

49. What is an **early** sign/symptom of tumor lysis syndrome? *(781)*
    1. Anuria
    2. Muscle weakness
    3. Paresthesias
    4. Tetany

50. What is the **most** effective regimen to manage
    the patient's cancer pain? *(784)*
    1. Patient-controlled analgesia
    2. Bolus dose for breakthrough pain
    3. Round-the-clock, fixed dose
    4. As needed, based on assessment

CRITICAL THINKING ACTIVITIES

Activity 1

51. During a routine checkup, a 40-year-old man voices questions about his potential for developing colon cancer. He relates his concerns about the recent death of his maternal grandfather from colon cancer.

    a. Discuss how a family history of colon cancer affects the recommendations for screening examinations for this patient. *(764)*

    _____

    _____

    _____

    _____

    b. What preventive behaviors should be included in discussions with this patient? *(767)* _____

    _____

    _____

    _____

    _____

Activity 2

52. A 32-year-old patient is being treated with unsealed internal radiation for thyroid cancer. Identify precautions to reduce radiation exposure to staff members who care for this patient. *(776)*

    _____

    _____

    _____

    _____

    _____

    _____

    _____